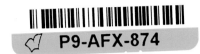
the ultimate workout log

an exercise diary and fitness guide
second edition

suzanne schlosberg

Houghton Mifflin Company
Boston • New York • 1998

For information about permission to reproduce
selections from this book, write to Permissions,
Houghton Mifflin Company, 215 Park Avenue South,
New York, New York 10003.

ISBN: 0-61813270-8

Anatomical diagram by Karen Kuchar
Design by Catharyn Tivy

Printed in the United States of America

QBP 10 9 8 7 6

To my family

Expert Contributors

Richard D. Ferkel, M.D., clinical instructor of orthopedic surgery, UCLA School of Medicine; attending physician, Southern California Orthopedic Institute, Van Nuys, California

Susan Levy, M.S., R.D., nutrition consultant in New York City

Liz Neporent, M.A., fitness consultant certified by the American College of Sports Medicine, National Strength and Conditioning Association, American Council on Exercise, and National Academy of Sports Medicine

Elizabeth Somer, M.S., R.D., author of *Age-Proof Your Body* (William Morrow, 1998) and *Food and Mood* (Henry Holt, 1995); nutrition consultant to ABC's *Good Morning America*

contents

Introduction: Why Keep a Log?   7

How to Use Your Log   10

Fitness Guide   17

    Cardio Exercise   18

    Strength Training   26

    Health Club Hints   36

    All About Injuries   42

    Fueling Up   47

Workout Diary   55

How Many Calories Do You Burn?   153

Workout Ratings: The Big Picture   154

Personal Records   155

Six-month Wrap-up   156

Resources   157

Sources   158

Acknowledgments   160

introduction

Why Keep a Log?

I've never been a fan of diaries. Back in high school, our English teacher made us record our thoughts and feelings in a journal, but the assignment seemed like a hassle so I ignored it. Then I paid: To pass the class, I had to spend one very tedious weekend faking an entire semester's worth of diary entries.

Somehow, though, I've always loved keeping an exercise log. I have 15 logs in my closet, dating back to 1988. Tracking my workouts gives me a sense of purpose when I'm riding my bike or lifting weights at the gym. It inspires me to push a little harder on some days and reminds me to back off when I'm tired. My log gives me confidence and a feeling of accomplishment.

For me, the benefits of keeping a training diary can be summed up in two words: Death Ride. The Death Ride is a 130-mile cycling event in Northern California that includes five steep mountain passes and pretty much lives up to its name. Every spring I sign up for the ride, and then I worry: Can I really get in shape for this thing when I've barely cycled all winter and a measly little hill leaves me winded?

But then I excavate my logs from the closet and find the answer in my illegible scribbles: Of course I can. Every year I start with 15-mile training rides; every year I finish the Death Ride. (Okay, every year but one; let's not discuss that.) When the big day comes and I'm scarfing down ice cream sandwiches at the top of the fifth mountain pass, I feel pretty darn good. And when I go home and write "Death Ride—finished strong!" in my log, success seems that much sweeter.

Achieving Your Goals

Whether you're aiming to lose 10 pounds, do 20 pushups, or compete in a triathlon, your log will help you get results. It will reveal patterns in your workouts and help you discover how much exercise — and how much rest — works best for you.

This log has several designated spaces for recording your goals — goals for the next six months and more specific objectives for each week. You'll accomplish a lot more if you have a plan than if you wander aimlessly through your workouts.

Top athletes know this well. Masters swim champion Alex Kostich used to write his goals on his kickboard; now he tapes them to his bathroom mirror. Amy Rudolph, the American record-holder in the 5,000 meter run, jots her long-term goals in the back of her training log. "If I have disappointments along the way," she says, " it helps me realize there are things farther down the road to look forward to."

Weightlifter Pete Kelley, a 1996 Olympian, keeps a picture of the Olympic rings next to his bed. "I wake up every morning and see those rings and it reminds me what I'm here for," Kelley says. "I'm a pretty lazy guy, so otherwise I probably wouldn't work out."

The word "lazy" doesn't exactly apply to a guy who can clean and jerk 424 pounds, but Kelley has a point. It's hard for anyone — accomplished athlete or complete novice — to stay motivated without a mission. Research confirms the importance of setting concrete workout goals. In a three-month study conducted at Miami University in Ohio, researchers told a group of exercisers that their goal was to increase by 20 percent the number of abdominal crunches they could do; they told a second group simply, "Do your best." Not surprisingly, the group with the concrete goal performed a significant 10 percent better than their rudderless peers.

A Diary After All

It's funny: Although I've never had the discipline to keep a personal diary, my training logs have turned out to serve a similar purpose. Sure, they're mostly filled with numbers and dates and phrases like "awesome run" or "totally zonked." But I always note which friends I exercise with, and I take my workout diary on vacations. So when I flip back through my logs, as I do on occasion, I see more than improvements in my bench press. I see a chronicle of my life.

With a glance at my logs I remember getting attacked by mosquitoes while cycling in Texas. I remember the boyfriend who convinced me to run around the town of Yerington, Nevada, carrying a 50-pound sack of chicken feed on my shoulders. (No joke; it's a quadrennial event called the Great American Sack Race.) I remember my trip to the Micronesian island of Yap, where I happened upon the island's only gym — a tin shack where the locals hoist rusty barbells while chewing betel nut, a mild narcotic that stains your teeth red. According to my log, I had a great chest and shoulder workout that day. I'm glad I decided to record it.

What's New in the Second Edition

If you used the first edition of this log, you'll notice some improvements. Now you have space for daily nutrition notes, plus a daily box to record whether you stretched. The second edition is filled with new training tips based on current research, along with a new batch of fun sports slang and new inspirational quotes from world-class athletes. The Fitness Guide has been updated, too, reflecting the latest thinking about body-fat testing, sports nutrition, and other exercise topics. You'll find the new question-and-answer format handy as well. The Resources section on page 157 lists a number of excellent books that can supplement the information here.

how to use your log

If you're new to exercise and this log seems as confusing as a tax form, skip ahead to the Fitness Guide before you read this section. But if you're already familiar with common workout terms—sets, reps, cardio, target heart rate—stay right where you are.

This is your log; you can make as many or as few notes as you want. The amount of information you write will probably vary over time. You may go through phases when you want to track every aspect of your exercise program, from your resting heart rate to what you ate before each workout to what the weather was like. At other times, you may simply want to write, "Went biking."

Even if you record minimal information, it's a good idea to write *something* every day—and that includes days you don't exercise. This way, when you look back, you'll be able to distinguish between days you rested and days you were sick or injured. You'll have more clues as to how much training works best for you.

When deciding what type of notes to make in your log, consider the experience of runner Matt Giusto, a 1996 Olympian in the 5,000 meters. "I used to put way too much information in my log," he says. "I'd even write down which of my five pairs of shoes I wore and track how much mileage I put on each shoe." Eventually, he says, he found the note-taking tedious and stopped recording his workouts altogether. "I figured I'd been doing it for so long that I could just rely on my common sense."

But abandoning his log wasn't the solution, either. "I'd get to a race and think, 'Wait, how did I train last year? How many rest days did I take?' Now, Giusto has found a happy medium, logging how far he ran, how fast he ran, and how he felt. "I keep it simple," he says. "But it's helpful to have my log going again."

Here's a look at the various sections of this log, along with sample ways of recording your workouts. Eventually, you'll create your own shorthand system.

Goals for the Next Six Months

This page, located on the inside front cover of the book, is where you consider the big picture: what you'd like to accomplish over the next six months. You can set separate goals for cardiovascular fitness, strength training, and nutrition, along with broader goals in the "Overall goals" section.

How high you reach may depend on your personality. Some people get fired up by goals that seem far-fetched; they rise to the occasion and perform extraordinarily well. Other people respond better to goals that are more down to earth. In one study, researchers gave their subjects a seemingly impossible goal: improve their sit-up performance by 60 repetitions over three months. Thirty percent of the subjects actually met the goal. Others, however, lost motivation to train; they were demoralized because they felt the goal was way out of reach.

Figure out what type of goals work best for you. For most people, moderately difficult goals—those that are challenging but well within your capabilities—seem to work well. Whatever goals you set, don't be a slave to them. If your training isn't going according to plan, cut yourself some slack. Cross out the old goals and pencil in new ones.

Goals for the Week

Start each week by identifying a mission. You can set these weekly goals in a variety of ways. For instance, you can plan in terms of distance ("Bike 60 miles"), time ("Walk 30 minutes a day"), or number of sessions ("Lift weights three times"). Remember that not all goals involve numbers. You might aim to eat less saturated fat, hike more hills, or just enjoy your workouts more. If you plan to push yourself hard some weeks, be sure to balance out your program with weeks of easy workouts, too.

Cardio Exercise

In this section you can record three different activities, your times, and the distance you covered. There's also room to make additional notes, such as how you felt after your workout, who you exercised with, or what type of terrain you covered. Say you rode the stationary bike for 15 minutes on level 4 and then jogged on the treadmill for 15 minutes at 5.5 mph. You might write:

CARDIO EXERCISE	TIME/DISTANCE	NOTES
bike	15 min. (L4)	felt energized!
treadmill	15 jog (5.5 mph)	

If you ran 4 miles with Tina at Balboa Park in 35:12 and felt especially strong on the hills, you might write:

CARDIO EXERCISE	TIME/DISTANCE	NOTES
run w/Tina	35:12 / 4 mi., hilly	flew up the hills!

Say you checked your resting heart rate the morning after a hard run and found it to be 68 beats per minute, 8 beats higher than usual. You felt tired and decided to take a yoga class instead of step aerobics.

CARDIO EXERCISE	TIME/DISTANCE	NOTES
yoga	1 hr.	RHR 68 — high;
		still tired from big run;
		no step!

Strength Training

In this section you can record your strength-training exercises, including how much weight you lifted and the number of sets and repetitions you performed. If you're a beginner, it's especially helpful to write down the names of the exercises. Many novices learn how to perform a routine without knowing which muscles each move is intended to strengthen. Writing down "lat pulldown" will reinforce the notion that the exercise strengthens your back muscles.

If you completed 3 sets of 10 reps using 80 pounds on the chest press machine, you might write:

STRENGTH TRAINING	WT.	SETS	REPS	NUTRITION NOTES
chest press	80	3	10	

Say you performed 3 sets of leg extensions: In the first set you did 12 reps with 75 pounds; the second, 10 reps with 90 pounds; the third, 5 reps with 105 pounds. You might write:

STRENGTH TRAINING	WT.	SETS	REPS	NUTRITION NOTES
leg ext.	75,90,105	3	12,10,5	

If you did 2 sets of 25 abdominal crunches on an incline board, 2 sets of 20 reverse crunches, and then 2 sets of 15 ab crunches with a twist, you might write:

STRENGTH TRAINING	WT.	SETS	REPS	NUTRITION NOTES
crunches (inc.)	—	2	25	
rev. crunches	—	2	20	
cr. w/twist	—	2	15	

Daily Rating

The Daily Rating is a measure of your intensity, not your success. Rate your workouts on a scale from 1 to 5 — not in terms of how far you went or how many calories you burned, but in terms of how hard you pushed your body. A 1 rating would be a very easy day; a 5 would be a killer workout. Shoot for a healthy mix of numbers. Log a 0 for days you don't exercise.

Each week, transfer your daily ratings to the chart on page 154 titled "Workout Ratings: The Big Picture." A glance at this chart will give you insight into your training. You might notice, for instance, that it's been two weeks since you took a day off. Or maybe it's been two weeks since you worked out at all!

Stretching

This box is new to the second edition. Check it on the days you perform flexibility exercises. Just remember: Stretching isn't a warm-up. Always stretch *after* you have warmed up your muscles with at least 10 minutes of cardiovascular exercise.

Nutrition Notes

In this box, also new to the second edition, you can track your eating habits. Rather than record every calorie you ingest, try focusing on one or two nutrition goals at a time. For instance, note how many fruit and vegetable servings you ate in a day or how much water you drank. If you're trying to lose weight, you might want to record a particularly healthy substitution, like "ate turkey sandwich instead of Big Mac."

To see how your eating habits affect your exercise performance, you might want to record what you eat before your workout. Over the course of a few weeks, look for any patterns. Maybe you tend to finish stronger on a two-hour bike ride when you eat a bagel with peanut butter than when you eat a plain bagel. Or maybe you perform better when you eat half an hour before a tennis match than when you eat two hours before.

Weekly Wrap-up

Here's your chance to look back at the week you just completed. Recording how much you accomplished one week can give you inspiration as you start the next.

■ *Weekly rating:* This needn't be a precise average of your daily ratings, but use this 1 to 5 scale to record how hard you pushed your body during the week. Transfer your weekly ratings to the chart on page 154.

■ *Goals:* It's easy to set goals, but it's even easier to forget you ever did. This section will keep you honest, forcing you to look back at the goals you set the previous Monday. If you consistently fall short, perhaps you have unrealistic expectations. On the other hand, if you frequently exceed your goals, perhaps you need more of a challenge.

■ *Cardio Notes:* Assess your week as a whole and record whether you felt strong or not up to par. You may want to note how many total hours you spent doing cardio exercise. Next to Total Sessions you can note how many days you exercised.

■ *Strength Notes:* Jot down anything significant that happened on the weight-training front. In the Total Sessions space, note how many times you lifted weights. If you do a split routine (working different muscles on different days), you may want to use the space above to record how many days you worked each muscle group or body area. For instance, if you did two upper-body workouts but worked your legs only once, you might note: "upper: 2, lower: 1."

■ *Nutrition Notes:* Record any patterns in your eating habits over the week. Maybe you chose nutritious snacks all week. Maybe you ate breakfast consistently or ate plenty of fruits and veggies.

■ *Stretching:* Flip back through the week and count how many days you stretched.

fitness guide

cardio exercise

Whether you're exercising to live longer, lose weight, or compete in a marathon, you're doing your body a lot of good. Regular cardiovascular workouts strengthen your heart, so it can pump more blood with each beat, and also strengthen your lungs, so you can take in more air with each breath. As a result, your stamina increases and you can get through your workouts—and your daily life—with less effort and wear and tear on your body. Cardio exercise has been shown to lower blood pressure and improve blood cholesterol levels and it is associated with a reduced risk for heart disease, diabetes, and colon cancer. What's more, moderate exercise can strengthen your immune system and help relieve anxiety and depression.

There's no limit to the ways you can increase your cardiovascular fitness. You can walk, jog, swim, bike, skate, hike, climb stairs, even go dancing. Here are the answers to some common questions about cardio exercise.

For good health, how often and how long do I need to exercise?

There's no magic number; exercise scientists haven't determined precisely how much cardiovascular exercise it takes to have positive impact your health. But health benefits do seem to be proportional to the amount of activity you do. In other words, the more the better—up to a point.

The Surgeon General's report *Physical Activity and Health* recommends at least 30 minutes of exercise on most days of the week. The report's definition of exercise includes brisk walking, lawn mowing, even raking leaves—any activity that gets you slightly winded. And according to the report, you need not perform these 30 minutes of exercise consecutively; two 15-minute walks or three 10-minute walks will suffice.

But these are minimum numbers, and they apply primarily to people who don't exercise at all. Research indicates that people who exercise longer and harder will benefit more. Be aware, however, that too much exercise can actually harm your health. Overtraining can suppress your immune system, leaving you at greater risk for infections and colds; plus, overtaxing your body can lead to muscle, joint, and tissue injuries. Rest is just as important to good health as exercise. Be sure to increase your cardiovascular workouts gradually, and listen to your body.

How much exercise does it take to lose weight?

Again, there's no formula. Weight loss depends on a lot of things, including how much you eat and your body's metabolism. But it's probably safe to say that if your goal is to slim down, gardening a few days a week isn't going to cut it. A landmark study recently looked at the exercise habits of weight-loss success stories—men and women who lost an average of 66 pounds and kept the weight off for an average of five years. Virtually everyone in the study reported exercising regularly and more than half of the subjects reported burning at least 2,000 calories per week through exercise. That's roughly the equivalent of jogging for 40 minutes or walking for an hour five days a week. To lose weight and keep it off, experts generally recommend burning at least 1,000 calories per week through exercise. (See the chart on page 153 to estimate how many calories you burn through different activities.)

If you're trying to lose weight, a registered dietitian can help you determine approximately how many calories you should burn through exercise each day or each week and how many calories you should eat. Typically, permanent weight loss requires both regular exercise and attention to your eating habits.

How hard should I push myself?

If you're exercising simply to improve your health, forget about the old saying, "No pain, no gain." Exercise does not have to hurt in order to be good for you. On the other hand, to challenge your cardiovascular system, you do need to take more than a leisurely stroll. The simplest way to find the middle ground is to take the talk test. If you're too breathless to say hello to the guy on the treadmill next to you, you're pushing too hard. If you're comfortable enough to belt out the national anthem, you're not pushing hard enough.

Of course, if you want to get significantly stronger and faster—for competition or personal satisfaction—you'll need to push to the point of discomfort at times. (See "What is your target heart zone?" below for details.) But always pay attention to how you feel and use common sense. For the first five to ten minutes of every workout, warm up at a very easy pace. If at any time you feel dizzy, faint, or nauseous, slow down and then stop. See your doctor if any of these symptoms persist.

What is your target heart zone?

Although the talk test is a valid way to gauge your exercise intensity, there's a more precise method: measuring your heart rate, the number of times your heart beats per minute. Your heart rate during exercise is an excellent indicator of the stress on your body. If your heart is beating too fast, you may be overtaxing your body. If your heart is barely thumping faster than it does when you're not exerting yourself, you may not get much benefit from your workout. Your target heart zone is a range of intensity levels generally considered safe and effective for exercise. The American College of Sports Medicine defines this zone as 50 to 85 percent of your maximum heart rate (the fastest your heart can beat).

However, this is an immensely wide range. Exercise at 50 percent of max feels a heckuva lot different from working out at 85 percent. If you're a beginner, stay at the low end of your target zone—in the 50 to 70 percent range—until this pace feels comfortable. Then you can start mixing in short stints at higher intensities. (For instance, you may want to alternate three minutes of walking with one minute of jogging.)

Unless you're a competitive athlete, there's no reason to work as high as 90 percent of your maximum. Even if you do compete or want to get as fit as possible, it's best to mix high-intensity workouts with slower-paced training sessions—or vary your pace within a workout. Even top athletes don't train as hard as they can all the time.

How do I know if I'm in my target zone?

To find your target zone, first determine your maximum heat rate. But don't do this by sprinting as hard as you can and then counting your heartbeats for one minute. You can estimate your maximum heart rate without moving. The simplest way is to subtract your age from 220. Then, to find your target zone, calculate 50 percent and 85 percent of this number.

Here's how a 35-year-old would do the calculations:

$$220 - 35 = 185$$

$$185 \times .85 = 157.25 \text{ high end} \qquad 185 \times .50 = 92.5 \text{ low end}$$

So if you're 35, your heart rate should stay somewhere between 93 and 157 beats per minute when you exercise. Keep in mind that this formula provides only an estimate of your maximum heart rate. Your true max might be as much as 15 beats higher or lower. Also, this formula tends to be most accurate for activities in which your feet hit the ground. When you ride a bike, your maximum heartbeat is about 5 beats slower than when you run; when you swim, your max might be a full 10 beats slower.

How do I measure my heart rate?

The low-tech way is to take your pulse, on your wrist or your neck. For the wrist method, lightly press your first two fingers (not your thumb) on the artery that's close to the base of your thumb and feel the thumping. For the neck method, place your fingers on the artery that runs straight down from the corner of your eye just underneath your chin.

Whichever method you choose, count the number of beats for 15 seconds and multiply the number by 4. You now have your heart rate. It's a good idea to stop exercising completely to get an accurate count. If you take your pulse while you're walking, you may end up counting your footsteps instead of your heartbeats.

If you don't want to interrupt your workout to take your pulse—and if you want more accuracy — you can wear a heart-rate monitor that straps around your chest. A chest monitor reads your heart's electrical activity and transmits the information to a receiver that you wear on your wrist. (Monitors that clip onto your ear or fingertip tend to be less accurate.) If you memorize your target zone, you can glance at your wrist and know instantly whether your heart rate is in the right range. Some monitors come with an alarm that can be set to beep when you exceed or fall below your target zone. Monitors cost about $80 to $200.

How often should I check my heart rate?

If you're a beginner, it's a good idea to check your heart rate — or at least take the talk test — a couple of times each workout. Once you get a feel for how your body reacts to exercise, you can do a pulse check every few weeks. Knowing your heart rate can keep you motivated and can help you design or redesign your exercise program. For instance, your goal might be to ride the stationary bike for 20 minutes at level 6; but if your heart rate is too high at that level, you may need to go down a few notches. On the other hand, if your heart rate is too low, you may want to crank up your intensity.

Monitoring your heart rate periodically — and charting it in your log — can give you an idea of how you're improving. Let's say you can run 3 miles in 30 minutes while maintaining a heart rate of 140. A few months later you may be able to cover a lot more ground — maybe 3.3 miles — in the same amount of time at the same heart rate. You know you have become more fit when you can accomplish more work without putting more stress on your body.

You also know you're improving when you experience a decrease in your resting heart rate, the number of times your heart beats per minute when you're sitting still. Top athletes in endurance sports have resting heart rates as low as 30 or 40 beats per minute. Someone who doesn't exercise at all may have a resting heart rate of 80 beats per minute. In other words, a couch potato's heart may have to work twice as hard to pump the same amount of blood as an elite athlete's. Keep in mind that your heart rate is in part genetically determined. If your resting heart rate is 60 and your friend's is 55, this doesn't necessarily mean that your friend is in better shape.

Yet another way to track your improvement is to measure your recovery heart rate, how quickly your heart slows down after a workout. For instance, check your heart rate right after you've run two miles and then one minute later. Perform this test after two months of training and see if your heart rate drops more quickly.

Will I burn more fat if I exercise at a slow pace?

No, that's a myth. When you exercise at a slow place, a greater *percentage* of the calories you burn comes from stored fat. (No matter what your pace, you always burn some fat and some carbohydrate.) However, the slower you exercise, the fewer calories you burn, so it doesn't matter that a greater percentage of those calories comes from fat. For weight loss, what really matters is the total number of calories you burn.

Let's say you walk on a treadmill for a half hour at a leisurely 20-minutes-per-mile pace. If you weigh 180 pounds, you'll burn about 172 calories. If you push harder and jog at a 10-minute-mile-pace, you'll burn about 440 calories. But this doesn't necessarily mean that faster is better. If you're new to exercise, you probably won't be able to sustain a 10-minute-mile pace for very long (and you may be so uncomfortable that you quit working out altogether). A better strategy may be to slow down so you can exercise longer, burn more calories, and have more fun.

Are the calorie counts on cardio machines accurate?

The numbers that flash on stationary bikes, stairclimbers, and other machines are only estimates (as are the numbers in the chart on page 153). Some machines are off by as much as 20 percent, and even the best ones can't factor in your metabolism, which greatly affects how many calories you burn during exercise.

Calorie counts are most accurate when you're using proper form on the machines. If you're clenching the side rails on the treadmill or leaning forward on the stairclimber, you're not burning nearly as many calories as the machine says you are.

What are the most effective cardio machines?

Despite the hype you may see on TV infomercials or read in magazine ads, no single machine is better than all the rest. You can get fit on just about any machine, as long as you use it regularly and push yourself hard enough.

To stay motivated and avoid overuse injuries, it's a good idea to vary the machines you use. For instance, you might want to do 20 minutes on the stairclimber, which emphasizes the front thigh muscles, and then 20 minutes on the recumbent bike, which places more emphasis on your rear thigh muscles and less stress on your back.

Here are key tips for using the most popular machines.

Stairclimber

■ Stand up straight and place your hands lightly on the machine in front of you or on the side railings. Don't cheat by hugging the console or turning your palms around and locking your elbows. These tactics deprive your butt and leg muscles of a great workout and they can greatly reduce the number of calories you burn. Locking your elbows can also lead to tendinitis in your arms and elbows.

■ Don't let the pedals sink all the way to the floor or rise as far as they can. Taking very deep steps can aggravate your lower back and knees. However, taking very short, choppy strokes reduces the number of calories you burn. Find a happy medium.

Stationary Bike (Upright and Recumbent)

■ Adjust the seat so that when your leg straightens to the farthest point in your pedal stroke, your knee is slightly bent. This position protects your knees.

■ Tighten the toe straps so they fit snugly around your shoes. As you pedal, think of creating a circle with the balls of your feet instead of just pushing down on the pedals. You'll save energy this way.

Treadmill

■ Never turn the machine on or off while standing on the belt. Instead, start with one foot on either side of the belt, turn on the machine, and then step onto the moving platform. Grasp the handrails momentarily, until you catch your balance.

■ Keep your chest up and your chin level and take comfortable, not exaggerated, strides. Try not to grab the handrails; you'll move more naturally and burn more calories if you let your arms swing freely.

Rowing Machine

■ Remember that rowing is a three-part motion: First push with your legs, then pull with your upper body, then bring your arms into your chest. With practice, you'll move fluidly from one part to the next.

■ Keep your back straight the whole time and don't lock your knees when you straighten your legs.

Cross-Country Skier

■ Start by mastering the leg movements; add the arm swing later. Cut yourself some slack when you to learn how to use this machine. You may need two or three sessions to get the hang of it.

■ Vary your stride length to work different muscle groups. Longer strokes bring your butt muscles more into play than shorter, more clipped strides, which emphasize your thighs.

Elliptical Trainer

■ Try pedaling your legs both forward and backward. The forward motion relies more on your glutes (butt muscles) and quadriceps (front thigh muscles); pedaling backward uses more hamstrings (rear thighs).

■ Don't lean forward or hug the arm rails. This isn't good for your lower back and it decreases the number of calories you burn.

strength training

These days everyone and their mother is lifting weights — and for good reason, especially for Mom. Between ages 35 and 40, most women gradually start losing bone mass. Weight training can slow this loss dramatically and perhaps even reverse it. Men aren't immune to bone loss, either (although, for hormonal reasons, it happens to them later in life). Maintaining strong bones will keep you standing tall rather than hunched over and help prevent osteoporosis, the brittle bone disease that causes millions of fractures each year.

Of course, weight training has more obvious — and immediate — benefits: You'll firm up your body and strengthen your muscles. You'll look healthier, feel more energetic, and have more oomph when you play basketball, lift your kids, or haul out the garbage.

Lifting weights can even help you lose weight and keep it off. If you try to slim down through dieting alone, you'll lose muscle along with fat. As a result, your metabolism may slow down, making it tougher to keep off the weight. But if you include weight training in your program, you'll maintain and perhaps increase your muscle mass and thereby keep your metabolism humming along.

This section answers common questions about lifting weights.

Do I really need to learn the names of my muscles?

Yes! Knowing your delts from your lats will help you learn the purpose of the exercises you perform. For instance, you'll understand that the lat pulldown is a back exercise, not an arm exercise, as many beginners mistakenly think. By knowing which exercises target which muscle groups, you can design a more balanced workout program. Plus, when someone at the gym says, "I worked quads and glutes today," you won't feel like you need an interpreter. The drawing on page 27 points out the major muscles of your body.

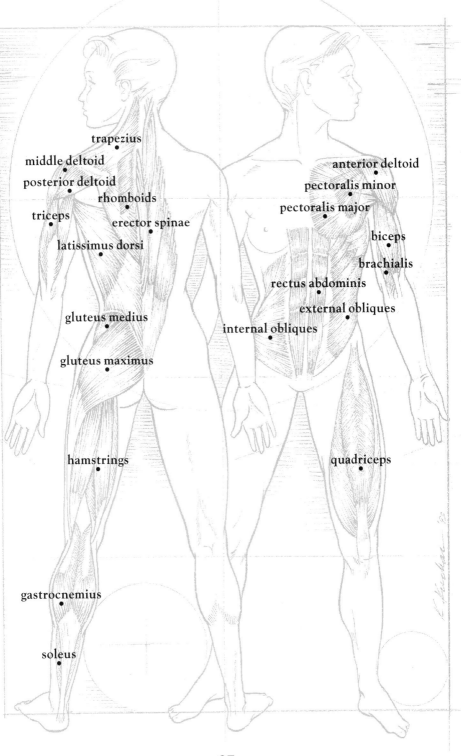

trapezius

middle deltoid

posterior deltoid

rhomboids

triceps

erector spinae

latissimus dorsi

gluteus medius

gluteus maximus

hamstrings

gastrocnemius

soleus

anterior deltoid

pectoralis minor

pectoralis major

biceps

brachialis

rectus abdominis

external obliques

internal obliques

quadriceps

Should I use free weights or machines?

Try both. You might think that machines are best for beginners and free weights (barbells and dumbbells) are only for serious lifters, but that's not the case. Free weights are perfectly safe for most novices, and they vastly expand your weight-training options. For instance, most gyms have only one biceps machine, but with free weights you can train your biceps a dozen or more different ways. At the same time, certain muscle groups—such as your back, calves, and rear thighs—are more easily trained with machines.

The more equipment you learn how to use, the better. You may find that you prefer machines for triceps exercises but free weights for your shoulders. You may end up staying at a hotel that only has free weights, so you'll need to know how to get a good workout without machines. Here's a closer look at the most common categories of strength-training equipment.

■ Weight machines

Machines do have one clear advantage for beginners: They require less co-ordination than free weights. Machines support your body and take you through a set motion, so you're more likely to use good form. Plus, there's no danger of dropping a barbell on you or anyone else.

Consider the shoulder press machine: You sit on a padded chairlike con-traption, grab a set of handles near your shoulders, then push the handles up. The free-weight version of this exercise involves essentially the same motion: You press up a barbell or a set of dumbbells. But the free weight exercises are tougher because you have to hoist the weights into position and keep them balanced as you push them upward. You also must rely on your abdominal and back muscles to keep your body still.

Machines are particularly convenient if you want to do a fast-paced workout or you're in a hurry. To change the weight, all you have to do is place a pin in a hole. With some free-weight exercises, you have to pile weight plates on and off, which can be time-consuming.

■ Free Weights

For reasons explained above, free-weight exercises are more difficult to perform correctly than machine exercises. On the other hand, free weights are less constricting than machines. Everyone's body is different, and yours may not feel comfortable going through the precise motion taken by that shoulder-press machine.

Dumbbells are particularly versatile. They allow each side of your body to move the way it does naturally. They also force your weaker side to do its share of the work; on a machine your stronger side can easily take over.

If you plan to work out at home, free weights may be your best option. You can do literally hundreds of exercises with a set of dumbbells. Machines aren't nearly as versatile.

■ Rubber Tubing

For convenience, nothing beats a rubber tube or band. You can use it at home or at the office or slip it in your luggage on vacation. If you buy a tube with handles and a door attachment, you can mimic just about every free-weight and machine exercise. You can learn a variety of band exercises by taking a body sculpting class at your gym or by watching the instructional videos that come with most bands.

Still, exercise bands do have their drawbacks. For one thing, you can't measure how much work you're doing. You know you've improved when you graduate from curling a 25-pound barbell to a 30-pounder. But with a band, you can't gauge your progress with much precision. Also, you can't build as much power with bands as you can with weights. Pulling on a band certainly can strengthen and tone your muscles, but to reach your potential, you'll have to hit the weight room.

Which exercises should I do?

Start by having a trainer teach you one or two exercises for each muscle group. (See "Health Club Hints" for tips on hiring a qualified trainer.) Practice your routine for a month or two before you learn new moves. If you take on too many new exercises at once, you may feel overwhelmed and forget how to perform them properly. Once you get the hang of things, you can expand your repertoire and vary your workouts.

Make sure that your routine is balanced. In other words, when you work one muscle group, you also need to exercise the muscle that works opposite to it. For instance, it's important to give your quadriceps (front thighs) and hamstrings (rear thighs) equal time. Many people focus on the muscle groups they see in the mirror, such as the chest, shoulders, and biceps, while neglecting less obvious muscles such as the lower back and butt muscles.

You don't need to work all of your muscle groups on the same day (for details, see "How many days a week should I lift weights?" on page 32), but just make sure no group gets left behind. Muscle imbalances can lead to a variety of injuries. Use the Weekly Wrap-up section of your log to track whether you're giving each muscle group enough attention.

Does the order of my routine matter?

To some extent. The basic rule is to work your larger muscle groups before your smaller ones. For instance, perform chest exercises before triceps exercises. This is because your triceps (rear arm muscles) help out when you perform chest exercises such as the bench press or pushups. If your triceps are worn out before you get to the bench press, they won't be strong enough to do their job; as a result, your chest muscles won't get as good a workout. For the same reasons, work your back muscles before your biceps. As for your legs, perform multimuscle exercises (such as squats, lunges, and leg presses) before doing exercises that "isolate" individual leg muscles.

Beyond this basic rule, you can perform your exercises in any order. In fact, it's a good idea to mix up the order. This way, you can hit different muscles when you're fresh.

How much weight should I lift?

The amount of weight you should lift depends on your goals. If you're looking to build the strongest, largest muscles that your body type will allow, lift heavy enough weights so that your muscles poop out after 5 or fewer repetitions. If you're looking for more moderate results—increased strength and tone but not bulging muscles—lift weights that cause your muscles to fatigue after 8 to 15 repetitions. Your last few reps should be quite difficult. If you get to your fifteenth rep and feel you could perform a few more, lift a heavier weight (but not so heavy that you compromise good form). Performing more than 15 repetitions won't give you much more strength.

Women tend to lift less weight than they can handle for fear that they'll get too bulky. But that's not going to happen. The overwhelming majority of women don't have enough testosterone to develop huge muscles. Besides, female bodybuilders lift extremely heavy weights and train for hours a day to develop their physiques.

If you're a weight-training novice, spend a few weeks in the 10 to 15 repetitions range, even if your ultimate goal is to get huge. Your muscles need time to adjust. Gradually increase your weights and drop down to 6 to 8 reps, then increase the weight even further. Keep in mind that you don't need to perform the same number of reps for every exercise.

How many sets should I do?

If you're lifting weights purely for the health benefits, a single set of each exercise may suffice. (Still, it's a good idea to perform a warm-up set with very light weights.) But if you're intent on developing significant muscle tone and strength, you'll probably need to perform at least 3 to 5 sets per muscle group. (You could do 3 sets of one back exercise and then 2 sets of another.) Body-builders perform 20 or more sets per muscle group, working each muscle from a variety of angles.

How long should I rest between sets?

The heavier your weights, the longer you'll need to rest. If you're perform-ing 5 repetitions per set, you may need 3 or more minutes to recover between sets. But if you're using much lighter weights and performing, say, 12 reps, you may need only 30 seconds' rest.

One way to cut down on your rest periods is to alternate between exer-cises that work different muscle groups. In other words, you can go straight from a hamstring exercise to a back exercise to a chest exercise without resting because each muscle gets a break while you're working another.

How many days a week should I lift weights?

Work each muscle group two or three times a week, and never on consecutive days. Muscles need at least 48 hours to recover from a workout.

If you plan to do more than 3 sets per muscle group, you may want to do a "split" routine. This means you split your workout into parts, working different muscle groups on different days. For instance, you could train your upper body muscles on Mondays and Thursdays and your lower body and abdominal muscles on Tuesdays and Fridays. Or you could do a split routine called the push/pull. You split your pushing muscles (chest and triceps) from your pulling muscles (back and biceps). You can include your shoulder and lower-body muscles on either day, or work them on a third day.

The benefit of doing a split routine is that you can put all of your energy and concentration into a few muscle groups. If you tried to perform 5 sets per muscle group and work your entire body in a single workout, you'd be at the gym for hours. You'd probably get tired and distracted and give short shrift to the muscles you hit at the end of your workout.

Whether you want to lift weights two days a week or six, a trainer can help you design a workout that fits into your schedule and gets you the results you want.

How can I keep weightlifting from getting boring?

The more variety you include in your workouts, the better. Changing your routine around will keep you motivated and keep your muscles stimulated. If you do the same old routine all the time, your muscles will adapt to it and you may stop making progress. You can vary the amount of weight you lift, the number of reps and sets you perform, the amount of rest you take between sets, the number of exercises you do, the sequence of the exercises, and the type of equipment you use. Tracking this information in your log will remind you to keep varying your routine. Here are some additional ways to keep your workouts fresh.

■ Do a pyramid. That is, decrease the number of repetitions while you increase the weight. For instance, do 12 reps of an exercise, then 10 reps with a heavier weight, and then 8 reps with an even heavier weight.

■ Do super sets. To really tax a specific muscle group, perform consecutive exercises that work the same muscle without resting between exercises. For instance, do a set of pushups and then go straight to the chest press machine.

■ Do a circuit. Instead of doing three sets of an exercise before moving on to the next exercise, perform one set of each, then repeat the whole routine two more times. Take little or no rest between exercises and don't work the same muscle group in consecutive exercises. A circuit routine will get your heart pumping faster than a traditional weight routine and may burn more calories. However, because you're moving so quickly, you probably won't be able to lift as much weight. Many gyms have circuit training classes.

■ Do super-slow training. Take twice as long as you normally would to perform each repetition. Eliminating most of the momentum will make your muscles work harder.

How long will it take to see results?

The answer depends on your genetics, your starting point, and the type of routine you perform. If you're a novice, you may make a lot of progress in the first few weeks, although typically this is due more to increased coordination than strength. It may take several months for your muscles to get significantly bigger or stronger.

Be patient. Some bodies respond to weight training a lot more quickly than others. Even if your biceps aren't popping out of your sleeves right away, you'll probably feel stronger and more energetic within a few weeks.

How can I avoid getting injured while lifting weights?

If you use common sense and follow these suggestions, it's unlikely you'll get injured pumping iron.

■ Do a cardiovascular warm-up. Before you lift a barbell or push the handles on a weight machine, get the blood flowing through your muscles with 5 to 10 minutes on the stairclimber, rowing machine, or another cardio machine. If you don't have access to cardio equipment that involves your upper body, warm up your back, chest, shoulders, and arms by doing arm circles.

■ Don't lift more weight than your muscles can handle. Otherwise you'll end up using poor technique and relying on muscles that the exercise is not intended to work. For instance, if you have to arch your back during the bench press in order to push up the weight, you may end up with a back injury. You should be able to control the weight throughout each repetition.

■ Use good form. Learn the correct posture and technique for each exercise— how low to squat, how high to raise your arms, how to grip the bar, when to breathe. (For most exercises, you exhale when you lift or press the weight and inhale when you lower it. For exercises that expand your chest cavity, such as seated rows, it may feel more natural to inhale as you lift the weight and exhale as you release it.)

■ Adjust each machine to fit your body. Don't be intimidated by the levers and notches; adjusting machines is simpler than it looks. A trainer can show you how to make each machine comfortable for you. If you don't bother to make the adjustments, you could strain a muscle while reaching for a bar.

■ Bend from your knees—not your waist—when lifting weights off a rack or hoisting them off the floor. This posture will protect your back.

■ Carry weight plates with two hands and with your elbows bent. Also, keep the plates close to your body, not dangling down by your sides.

■ Use collars. Collars are cliplike devices that slide onto the end of barbells to keep the weight plates secure.

■ Ask for a spot. If you're trying a free-weight exercise for the first time or you're lifting a heavier weight than usual, ask someone to "spot" you. Your spotter should stand behind you, ready to help in case you can't complete a repetition on your own. Some exercises require the spotter to place his or her hands near the weights, while other exercises are spotted at the elbows or waist. Ask a trainer to teach you proper spotting technique, or watch people in the gym. Let your spotter know how many repetitions you're planning to perform and at what point you think you'll need help.

health club hints

A gym is a lot more than a room with machines and barbells and a snack bar that sells protein smoothies; it's a place where you can get motivated to work out and get educated about your health and fitness. But a health club is only as good as its staff and its programs. This section answers questions that may come to mind when you walk into a club.

How can I get a good deal on a gym membership?

First, realize that the club that gives you the best price may not always be the best one for you. If the cheapest club in town is a half hour from your house, chances are you won't show up regularly, so it may not be such a great deal after all. You're more likely to go to a club that's within 10 minutes of your home or office, so factor convenience into the price. Also, a more expensive club may offer more of the amenities you're looking for, such as child care, a sauna, or longer hours.

That said, don't just write a check for the first price a gym salesperson offers you. Many clubs will waive their initiation fee if you balk at paying it. And if you're catching a club when business is slow, like in the summer, you may be able to bargain down the monthly fee. If you have a friend who recently joined and paid less than the price you're being quoted, mention this fact to the salesperson. You might save yourself some money.

While it makes sense to bargain for the best possible deal, don't sign up for a three-year membership just because the monthly fee is lower than the one-year plan. Clubs go out of business all the time; there's no guarantee yours will be around in three years. Besides, your needs may change during that time.

How do I know if the gym has a qualified staff?

More and more clubs are hiring employees who are educated about health and fitness; still, some gyms like to save money by hiring people with hard bodies but no formal fitness background. Be sure to ask what credentials the gym requires of its various staff members.

Trainers are most likely to be qualified if they are certified by one of the major fitness organizations, including the American College of Sports Medicine (ACSM), the American Council on Exercise (ACE), the Aerobics and Fitness Association of America (AFAA), the National Academy of Sports Medicine (NASM), and the National Strength and Conditioning Association (NSCA).

Also check the qualifications of specialty staff members. Anyone who calls himself or herself a nutritionist should be a registered dietitian (R.D.). Massage therapists should be licensed. All members of a gym staff should be certified in CPR.

Should I hire a trainer?

Most clubs will give you one or two free training sessions when you join, but it's a great idea to pay for at least a few extra sessions. (You'll probably pay $30 to $50 per session.) Whether you're a flat-out beginner or a fitness veteran who's fallen off the wagon, a trainer can give you an infusion of motivation, along with new workout ideas and technical guidance.

Five sessions should be enough to get you started, but it's helpful to schedule tune-ups a few times a year. This way the trainer can check your form and update your routine.

How do I know if I have a good trainer?

Your trainer should be certified by one of the professional organizations listed above and should be able to give explanations in English rather than exercise jargon. (If your trainer says things like "this routine will result in muscle hypertrophy" rather than "you'll get bigger muscles," find a new trainer.) Look for a trainer whose personality meshes with yours; some trainers take the perky cheerleader approach while others prefer drill-sergeant tactics.

Your trainer should ask what your goals are and then design a program tailored to your needs. Ask why your trainer has chosen certain exercises for you and not others. If an exercise doesn't feel right to you, ask to learn a different move for the same muscle group.

Make sure the trainer teaches you the principles behind your workout program so that you feel independent when your sessions are over. You should know how much weight you're lifting, how many sets and repetitions you're performing, and how to adapt your routine as you get stronger. Learn how to adjust each machine by yourself and how to perform each exercise with good form. Bring your log to your sessions and jot down the names of the exercises, tips on how to perform them ("pull bar to chest, not stomach"), and how much weight you used. That outer thigh machine may seem simple to operate when your trainer is there giving you instructions, but when you're on your own, the contraption may suddenly seem as unfamiliar as a forklift.

Don't be intimidated by your trainer. Ask a lot of questions and trust your instincts. If you don't feel your trainer has enough knowledge, teaching skills, or enthusiasm, hire somebody else.

Should I have my fitness tested before I start exercising?

Yes. When you join a gym, you should be offered a fitness assessment—a series of tests to determine how fit and healthy you are. You'll get pinched, measured, weighed, and asked to perform several exercises. These tests can be valuable if they're done correctly; they'll help you set goals and give you a starting point from which to measure your progress. But beware: Some testing methods aren't accurate, and others are only as good as the person who administers the test.

Before giving you a test, the club should determine if you're healthy enough to take it. You should at least be given a questionnaire that asks about your medical history and lifestyle. If you have had any heart or lung problems—or if you're a man over age 40 or a woman over age 50—get checked out by a medical doctor before joining a gym. When a trainer designs your program, he or she should have as much information as possible about your fitness level and injury or health risks.

Fitness tests generally cover four areas: cardiovascular fitness, strength, flexibility, and body composition. Here's a brief look at each.

■ *Cardiovascular Endurance*

A health-club trainer typically will test the strength of your heart by giving you a submaximal test—a test that measures your heart rate when you're exercising at less than maximum effort. A common submax test involves a step platform: You step up and down on a platform for two to four minutes, then the tester takes your pulse for one minute. The more fit you are, the more quickly your heart rate will drop.

A more accurate gauge of your cardiovascular fitness is a graded exercise test on a treadmill or stationary bike. You'll exercise at a low intensity for a few minutes, then pick up the pace for a few more minutes, then crank up your intensity again. Throughout the test, which typically lasts 9 to 15 minutes, the tester will take your pulse and blood pressure. Your tester should explain the results of your test and use this information to help you design a cardiovascular workout program appropriate for your fitness level.

■ *Strength*

Ideally, a strength test should involve a variety of muscle groups. Some clubs use only a grip test; you squeeze a metal gadget with a spring attached to a gauge. The grip test has been shown to correlate fairly well with overall upper-body strength, but it won't tell you anything about your leg muscles.

More commonly, a trainer will have you perform exercises on a variety of strength-training machines to see how many repetitions you can perform at a certain weight. This is a safer way to assess your strength than testing the maximum amount of weight you can lift once. Your trainer should use the results of your strength tests to design your weight-training program.

■ *Flexibility*

For flexibility, many clubs offer a sit-and-reach test: You sit with your legs out in front of you and reach for your toes. Ideally, the tester should measure the flexibility of other muscles and joints as well.

Learn which areas are particularly tight so you can work on those in your stretching program. Flexibility is an important and often neglected component of fitness. As you age, you typically lose flexibility, which can cause you to walk more stiffly and have more difficulty reaching for things.

■ Body Composition

A body composition test estimates how much of your body weight is composed of fat and how much is made of lean body mass—your bones, muscles, blood, tissues, and organs. Your body composition tells you more about your health than your weight does. That's because muscle weighs more per square inch than fat. A well-muscled athlete could be heavy according to the scale and yet be quite lean and healthy. On the other hand, a slim person who doesn't exercise may register a low weight on the scale but may actually have a greater percentage of body fat than an athlete who weighs a lot more.

How much body fat is too much? At your local health club you may be told that for a woman a healthy range is 18 to 25 percent; for a man, 10 to 17 percent. However, the latest research suggests that the standards should be relaxed a bit. It appears that a woman can have 35 percent body fat without being at increased risk for heart disease and certain cancers—as long as she exercises regularly and eats a nutritious diet. A man who has 25 percent body fat but is otherwise healthy, eating well, and exercising probably need not worry either.

What's more, when considering disease risk, total body fat should be taken in context with other measures, such as your cholesterol levels, blood pressure, and family history. The circumference of your waist may also be a helpful health indicator, probably more so than total body fat. Excess abdominal fat—the type that lies deep in your belly, clumped around your organs—has been correlated with increased risk for heart disease and other serious problems. (Fat on the hips and thighs, by contrast, doesn't seem to pose a health risk.) If your waist reaches 38 or 39 inches—whether you're male or female — see your doctor.

Keep in mind that having too little body fat can be unhealthy, too, particularly for women. Women who have less than about 18 percent body fat are at much greater risk for irregular periods, premature bone loss, and fractures. If you register below 18 percent on a body fat test, you may not be eating enough or you may be exercising too much. Have a registered dietitian analyze your eating habits.

So how do you know how much body fat you have? Most health clubs use a gadget called a skin-fold caliper. A caliper pinches your skin at specific points on your body, such as your triceps, hips, abdomen, and thighs. If the tester is experienced, the results can be fairly accurate, with a margin of error of 3.5 percent. But if he or she doesn't pinch precisely the right spots or the right amount of flesh, the margin of error can be as high as 10 percent or 12 percent.

Another popular method of testing body composition is bioelectrical impedance. You lie on your back while a signal is sent from an electrode on your foot to an electrode on your hand. The slower the signal travels, the more fat you have. An electrical current will move more quickly through lean tissue than fat because lean tissue contains more water (which conducts electricity). Since fat doesn't contain much water, it impedes the signal.

Bioelectrical impedance can be as accurate as skin-fold calipers, but the results also can be way off the mark. If you're dehydrated — and many people are without realizing it — the test may vastly overestimate your body fat. Also, different impedance manufacturers use different formulas to estimate body fat. Bioelectical impedance works best for people who have an average amount of muscle and fat; it's less accurate for those who have a lot of muscle or a lot of fat.

all about injuries

There's not much you can do to prevent a soccer opponent from kicking you in the thigh and sending you home with a nasty bruise; some sports injuries are simply out of your control. But the majority of pulls, sprains, and inflamed body parts are injuries you can prevent with smart training, proper gear, and common sense.

Be especially careful if you're new to exercise or if you're getting back in shape after a long layoff. You can't compensate for months — or years — of inactivity by suddenly jogging every day or climbing on every machine in the gym. This section answers questions about how to avoid injury and how to minimize the damage if you do get hurt. These answers apply to all kinds of exercise; for weightlifting safety tips, see page 34.

How can I keep from getting injured?

Be patient — with every aspect of your workout program. Don't rush from the locker room to an all-out sprint on the treadmill. Don't race through your weight-training repetitions. Don't make split-second decisions when you buy cross-training shoes. Don't expect to drop three pant sizes in three months. Give your body a chance to adjust to your exercise program and enjoy the process of getting in shape. The following tips can help keep you away from the physical therapist.

■ Warm up and cool down

Whether you're planning to jog 5 miles, lift weights, or play tennis, always begin your workout with at least 10 minutes of cardiovascular exercise at a slow pace. Warming up increases the blood flow to your muscles and makes them more pliable. Starting abruptly can leave you breathless and strain unprepared muscles.

End your workout the same way you started: with about 10 minutes of easy exercise. Your cool-down gives your heart a chance to adjust back to its normal pumping pace. If you stop suddenly, you risk nausea, dizziness, or fainting.

■ *Don't stretch cold muscles*

You may see some people start their workouts by touching their toes or performing other stretches; this is not a good idea. Don't stretch your muscles until after you have done a cardio warm-up; cold muscles are much more likely to tear than warm ones. In fact, you may be better off stretching after your entire workout than after your warm-up. Hold each stretch for at least 15 seconds without bouncing.

■ *Increase your training workload gradually*

Whatever your activity, start off at a comfortable pace, keep your workouts short, and progress gradually. A good guideline is the 10 percent rule: Don't increase your distance or time spent exercising by more than 10 percent each week. And don't increase your intensity and distance on the same day. In other words, either graduate from level 6 to level 7 on the stairclimber or add 5 minutes to your workout, but don't do both in the same workout.

■ *Take rest days*

If you want to get more fit, rest is just as important as working out. Taking days off gives your body a chance to recover and keeps you feeling fresh and motivated. How much rest you need depends on your body, your fitness level, and your activities. As a general rule, take at least one day off from cardiovascular exercise per week; with weight training, rest each muscle group at least 48 hours between workouts. If you find that you're getting weaker instead of stronger, chances are you need more rest. In addition to taking days off, alternate hard workouts with easy sessions. You also can save wear and tear on your body by cross-training—that is, varying your activities so you don't overuse any particular muscles or joints.

■ *Use proper form*

Whether you're running, climbing stairs, lifting weights, or doing step aerobics, learn the right technique from an expert. The more you repeat an incorrect motion, the more likely you are to get injured. Even subtle differences in form—such as gripping a barbell the wrong way or stepping too deeply on the stairclimber—can lead to significant injuries.

■ *Wear appropriate shoes*

Wearing worn-out shoes or the wrong shoes for your sport—or feet—can lead to heel pain, shin splints, tendinitis, and several other injuries. Don't do aerobics in tennis shoes or train for a 10k run in cross-trainers; shoes for each activity have special designs to accommodate the demands of that sport. Check to see if your feet roll inward (overpronate) or outward (oversupinate) and buy a shoe that's made for your foot type. Try on several pairs of shoes and make sure the pair you buy has enough support and cushioning. If you have persistent foot problems, consult an orthopedist or podiatrist to assess whether you need orthotics, corrective shoe inserts. They may be helpful if you have flat feet or an extremely high arch.

How do I know if I'm injured or just sore?

Sometimes exercise hurts; sore and stiff muscles are often part of the game. That's because in order to strengthen your muscles, you actually need to tear them down. When they rebuild themselves—in 4 to 48 hours, depending on the type of exercise—your muscles come back bigger and stronger. During this recovery period, you may feel some discomfort. That's normal—but intense pain isn't. It's important to distinguish normal soreness from pain that indicates injury.

You're probably injured if your pain persists for more than a few days and if it gets worse instead of better. Sharp pain is also a sign of injury. So is pain that's localized in a joint instead of in the surrounding muscles. Also beware if you have a new pain after doing the same old routine or if your pain seems out of proportion to your workouts. Other signs of injury are swelling, warmth, redness, numbness, weakness, and difficulty moving.

What should I do if I get injured?

The answer depends, of course, on the type and severity of your injury. Some injuries you can treat yourself; others require medical attention. Don't ignore an injury. Left untreated, a stress fracture, a tiny crack in your bone, can become a complete fracture and sideline you for months. Tendinitis can develop into a chronic problem that can end your running or tennis career.

One excellent guide to treating sports injuries is *The Return to Glory Days* (listed in Resources, on page 157). The book, cowritten by a physical therapist, explains how to treat forty common athletic injuries and describes signs that medical attention is in order. If you're not sure how severe your injury is, play it safe and see your doctor.

If your injury is relatively minor, such as a sprained ankle, you can use one of the basic rules for treating sports injuries: RICE. This acronym stands for Rest, Ice, Compression, Elevation. Rest your injured body part to prevent further damage; whatever your injury, do not try to "walk it off." Apply ice for 15 to 20 minutes three or four times a day for several days. Ice eases the pain and reduces the swelling and internal bleeding, limiting the amount of scar tissue formed and speeding up your recovery. (But beware: too much ice can cause blisters or tissue damage.) Compression — wrapping your injury with an elastic bandage — also helps reduce the swelling. The bandage should be tight enough that you feel some tension but not so tight that you cut off your circulation. Elevating your ankle or other injured area helps diminish the bleeding and swelling by allowing the blood to drain toward your heart.

What about heat? Heat won't relieve swelling but it can ease pain and muscle soreness. In general, don't put heat on an injury during the first 72 hours. After that time, you may want to use 10 minutes of heat followed by 10 minutes of ice — always in this order. (Ice before heat can actually increase the swelling.)

When can I start working out again?

You're ready to resume your old activities when you have no pain at all and when you can move the injured part normally again. If you start back too soon, you're likely to reinjure yourself, and this time you may cause more damage. When you do return, take it easy and ice your injury after each workout for a week or two. Remember that muscles atrophy quickly, so don't expect to be as strong as you were before you got hurt.

Injuries can be depressing, especially when they force you out of your regular exercise routine, but don't use your injury as an excuse to quit working out altogether. That will just make it tougher to get back in shape when you've healed. Instead, find an activity that doesn't affect your injury. If you strained your shoulder lifting weights, you can still use a number of leg machines and ride an exercise bike. If you have tendinitis in your knee from running, try swimming for a while.

Learn from your injury. If you got hurt by running too many miles or lifting too much weight, cut back this time. Your log can give you clues about where you went astray.

fueling up

Don't underestimate the power of food to help you exercise. If you're short on certain nutrients, changing your eating habits can take minutes off your 10k time, add yards to your swim workouts, help you concentrate on the tennis court, or add pounds to your bench press.

Of course, there's no shortage of advice—in magazines, in books, at health clubs, on TV—about how to eat right. Often, the advice is conflicting. First, high-carbohydrate diets are in; then high-protein eating is all the rage. And the market is flooded with powders, pills, and bars that claim to boost energy, burn fat, and build muscle. How do you know which claims are true?

This chapter outlines some nutrition basics, answering questions about what to eat to enhance your workouts. For more detailed nutrition information, consult the books listed under Resources on page 157.

When seeking out nutrition advice, remember this: Everyone's body is different. There are no absolute rules. Some people perform better when they eat more protein and less carbohydrate than others. Some people can scarf down a bagel minutes before a workout and feel fine; others prefer to wait an hour after eating before they exercise. Ultimately, you need to experiment with different eating plans and find what works best for you. (Always experiment *before* an athletic event or competition; the middle of a marathon is not a great time to test out a new sports drink.) There's room in your log for you to track how your eating habits affect your workouts.

How many calories should I eat per day?

The answer depends on your goals as well as your body weight, metabolism, and exercise habits. If you're at a desirable body weight and have plenty of energy, your calorie intake is right on; you don't need to take an exact count. But if you're gaining weight or feeling lethargic, you may want to count your calories and adjust upward or downward. Keep a food journal for a few days, making note of everything you eat and drink. (People often forget to record their beverages, which can contain a substantial number of calories.) Then add up the calories using one of the food values books found in bookstores or a nutrition computer program. Studies show that many people underestimate how much they eat while overestimating how much they exercise. Keeping track of this information in your log may prove eye-opening.

If your goal is to lose weight, don't go on a drastic calorie-reduction diet. You won't be able to fuel your workouts, you'll be low on essential nutrients, and you'll feel so deprived that you may swing the other direction and end up overeating. Plus, your body will sense that it's being starved and your metabolism will slow down, making it tougher to lose weight. A better strategy is to cut a few hundred calories per day and bump up your exercise. Don't aim to lose more than ½ pound to 1 pound per week.

It takes a deficit of about 3,500 calories to lose a pound of fat. In other words, you should lose 1 pound in a week if you cut 500 calories per day from your diet or burn an extra 500 calories per day through exercise. Or you could cut, say, 250 calories from your diet while burning an extra 250 calories through exercise. However, if you don't truly need to lose weight, the needle on the scale may not budge even if you do cut calories.

If losing weight is your goal, your best bet may be to consult a registered dietitian who can assess your current eating habits and help you come up with a plan tailored to your taste preferences, daily schedule, and exercise program. You may also want to see a dietitian if you suspect your eating habits are hampering your athletic performance — if, for instance, you're feeling sluggish, hungry, or lightheaded halfway through your workouts.

How much fat, carbohydrate, and protein should I eat?

Every diet book seems to have its own magic formula. Some books say a 10 percent fat diet is best; others promote the 40-30-30 plan — 40 percent carbohydrate, 30 percent protein, 30 percent fat. The reality is, there's no one-size-fits-all diet. Some people function best with a different nutrient balance than others. (However, most experts agree that getting 40 percent of your diet from carbohydrate is too low. See the carbohydrate section below for more details.)

The bottom line is, everyone needs a healthy mix of all three nutrients. Carbohydrates and fat are crucial for providing your body with energy, among other functions; protein is vital for building and repairing body tissues. (It can also be used for energy, but only as a last resort.) It's a good idea to combine all three nutrients at each meal. Here's a rundown of each nutrient and general guidelines on how much you need.

■ *Carbohydrate*

Carbs supply glucose, the fuel that runs your body. Your body stores very little carbohydrate, so you constantly have to restock. If your muscles don't get enough glucose, they'll tire easily and feel heavy. If your brain doesn't get enough, you'll feel sluggish and unmotivated. It's important to eat or drink carbs before you exercise, during a workout that lasts longer than an hour, and within two hours after your workout (although the sooner you refuel, the better).

Not all carbs are created equal. There are simple carbohydrates, such as sugar, soft drinks, hard candy, and refined fruit juices. These carbs are absorbed into your bloodstream quickly and can give you an immediate burst of energy, but they won't keep you satisfied for more than about a half hour, and they contain virtually no vitamins, minerals, or fiber.

Complex carbs, on the other hand, are metabolized more slowly and keep you satisfied longer, up to two hours. These include pasta, potatoes, rice, grains, fruits, vegetables, breads, and cereals. Simple carbohydrates can give you quick energy during a workout, but the majority of the carbs you eat throughout the day should be of the complex variety. The less processed the carbohydrate, the more fiber it's likely to have. (For instance, an orange has about 3 grams of fiber, whereas canned orange juice has none.)

How much carbohydrate you need in your diet depends on your body. Some people do fine getting 55 percent of their calories from carbs, while others may need 70 percent. One gram of carbohydrate contains 4 calories. So, if your yogurt contains 30 grams of carbohydrate and 170 calories, you know that 120 of the calories (30 grams at 4 calories per gram)—about 70 percent—come from carbs.

Despite what some high-protein advocates say, carbohydrates are not inherently fattening; they are, in fact, crucial as a fuel source, particularly for people who exercise regularly. If you don't eat enough carbohydrate, you'll experience chronic muscle fatigue, mood swings, and brain drain.

■ *Protein*

Protein supplies amino acids, which build and repair muscles, tendons, red blood cells, and enzymes. You can get protein both from animal and vegetable products. Animal protein sources include chicken, turkey, beef, seafood, fish, milk, yogurt, eggs, and cheese. Veggie sources of protein include beans, nuts, tofu, peas, and broccoli.

How much protein is enough? The average person needs about .8 grams per kilogram (2.2 pounds) of body weight. So, to figure out your protein needs, take your weight in pounds and divide by 2.2. Then multiply this number by .8. Let's say you weigh 150 pounds. Divide 150 by 2.2, and you get 68 kilograms. Multiply 68 by .8 and you get 54—the number of protein grams you need per day. You can exceed this number simply by eating a 3-ounce chicken breast (26 grams) and a cup of cottage cheese (31 grams).

If you exercise strenuously you may need more protein—1.2 to 1.8 grams per kilogram of body weight, depending on how intensely and frequently you work out. (You need extra protein to synthesize new cells, replacing the ones that break down during intense exercise.) However, many athletes mistakenly think that loading up on protein will build extra muscle; there's no evidence to support this theory. Besides, if you eat too much protein, it will be broken down to form fat. Also, if you fill your stomach with extra protein, you won't get enough carbohydrate to fuel your muscles. The typical American diet includes twice the amount of protein needed.

Experiment with how much protein keeps you satisfied, but in general, aim to get 15 percent to 20 percent of your calories from protein. Protein, like carbohydrate, contains 4 calories per gram.

■ *Fat*

Fat has become the enemy; many people try to eat as little fat as they possibly can. But in reality, fat is essential—for absorbing certain vitamins, maintaining your immune system, and keeping your skin moist, among other functions. Eliminating fat from your diet is not a good idea, either for good health or weight loss.

Most major health organizations recommend limiting fat to 30 percent of total calories, but the more important recommendation is limiting *saturated* fat to no more than 10 percent of calories, preferably less. There's a significant difference in fats. Saturated fat, found primarily in meat and dairy products, contributes to heart disease and some types of cancer. Whole-milk dairy products contain up to 80 percent saturated fat. On the other hand, unsaturated fat—found in nuts, avocados, olives, and most vegetable oils—has not been linked with disease.

Be aware, however, that all fats contain 9 calories per gram. So even healthy fats contain a lot of calories and should be eaten in moderation. Also know that a product labeled "98% fat-free" doesn't get 2 percent of its calories from fat. It gets 2 percent of its weight from fat. For instance, one brand of 2 percent milk contains 5 grams of fat per 140 calories; that's 45 fat calories (5 grams at 9 calories per gram), or 32 percent of the total calories.

Food labels can tell you what percent of calories come from fat—and how much of the fat is saturated.

Should I take a vitamin/mineral supplement?

Probably. There's no question that vitamins and minerals are crucial, especially for people who exercise. Vitamins and minerals don't give you energy because they don't supply calories, but they're involved in every one of your body's functions, including the crucial process of converting food into energy.

If you eat a balanced diet and enough calories (around 2,000 per day), you may get all of the vitamins and minerals you need. However, most of us don't eat enough fruits and vegetables, and even if you do make good food choices, it's tough to get enough of certain nutrients, such as vitamin E. Most of us fall short in some areas. For instance, many vegetarians are low in zinc and vitamin B12. Most women don't get enough calcium, iron, zinc, folic acid, and vitamin D.

So, for many people, a vitamin/mineral supplement is a good choice. Just don't count on supplements to make up for a junk-food diet. In some cases, it's not the vitamin or mineral itself that aids good health but rather the way these nutrients mingle with other components in food. Also, supplements don't contain fiber or phytochemicals, disease-fighting substances in foods that scientists are only beginning to understand. Aim to get the majority of your vitamins and minerals from food, especially fruits and veggies; no pill can make up for an inadequate diet.

How much water do I need to drink?

Water is the most important nutrient affecting athletic performance. When you exercise, you need water—and lots of it—to cool your body, carry nutrients to your cells, and carry waste to your kidneys. If you're chronically fatigued, you may be chronically dehydrated. Don't rely on thirst to tell you when to drink water; by the time your brain signals thirst, you may already be dehydrated. Dehydration can seriously impair your workouts, causing fatigue, dizziness, and headaches, among other symptoms. Dehydration can develop during a single workout or over several weeks.

You've probably heard you need to drink eight glasses of water per day, but if you exercise, you need several more. (By the way, your fluids don't have to come from water; juices, milk, and fruits and vegetables also are sources of fluids.) Drink before, during, and after exercise, and all day long. The American College of Sports Medicine recommends swigging 8 to 16 ounces of fluid before exercise, at least 4 ounces every 15 to 20 minutes while you're working out, and then at least 24 ounces afterward—more if it's hot.

The simplest way to tell if you're well hydrated is to check the color and quantity of your urine. If your urine is dark and scanty, you need to drink more fluids. If it's clear and plentiful, your body has returned to its normal water balance. If you're taking vitamin supplements, your urine may be dark; in that case, volume is a better indicator than color. Also, you can weigh yourself before and after exercise. For each pound of weight lost during a workout, you need to drink two cups of fluids.

Are sports drinks worth the money?

For years the conventional wisdom was that sports drinks are useful only when you exercise continuously for more than an hour. But recent research suggests these carb-spiked drinks can delay fatigue even in stop-and-go activities like basketball and tennis and perhaps even in activities that last less than an hour.

What's in these drinks that makes them better than plain old water? Sports drinks replenish fluids, just as water does, but they also offer two nutrients that water lacks: carbohydrate and sodium. By providing carbohydrate in an easily digestible form, sport drinks quickly deliver energy to your working muscles when they need it most.

Sodium, meanwhile, helps your body retain fluid, which in turn staves off dehydration. What's more, sodium drives your thirst mechanism, so you might end up drinking more of a sports drink than you would plain water. Plus, sports drinks taste good, so you might drink more fluid for that reason, too. It doesn't matter which brand you choose. Most of today's commercial sports drinks contain between 5 and 8 percent carbohydrate, which means they're absorbed into the bloodstream about as quickly as water. Juice and soda, on the other hand, contain 10 percent or more carbohydrate and therefore won't rehydrate you or fuel you up as effectively as a sports drink and may cause an upset stomach.

Can energy bars help my workouts?

Energy bars are helpful mostly because they're a convenient source of carbohydrate and calories. A typical energy bar contains the same amount of calories and carbs as two bananas, but it's tough to carry those bananas in your cycling jersey.

Know that bars contain different proportions of carbohydrate, protein, and fat. Some are high in carbs, containing about 250 calories and 40 to 45 grams of carbohydrate (about 70 to 80 percent of total calories). These can help fuel you up before a workout or during exercise, although after a workout it's best to eat real food.

At many health clubs you'll also see high-protein bars, which contain up to 30 grams of protein, two to four times as much protein as other bars. These bars may keep you satisfied longer than the high-carb variety, but they won't provide energy as quickly and won't replenish your carbohydrate stores as well. The same goes for bars that contain a higher percentage of fat.

Is it a bad idea to eat before a workout?

No, it's important! Sure, if you eat too much, you may get an upset stomach, but if you haven't eaten for hours, you'll run out of gas. Even if you exercise first thing in the morning, it's a good idea to at least drink something high in carbohydrate, such as orange juice. (While you sleep, your body is burning plenty of calories, and in the morning, your blood sugar will be low.)

If you're going for a long workout, you can increase your stamina by eating or drinking 100 to 300 calories of carbohydrate per hour. That would be equivalent to a sports bar, a couple of bananas, a bagel, an energy gel, or two cups of a sports drink.

How soon after a workout should I eat?

As soon as possible. Some people avoid eating right after a workout because they think they'll ruin everything by eating the calories they just burned. That's a counterproductive strategy. The sooner you eat after a workout, the faster you'll recover. Within the first two hours (sooner really is better), eat .5 grams of carbohydrate per pound of body weight. If you weigh 150 pounds, you need about 75 grams of carbohydrate—300 calories (since each gram of carbohydrate contains 4 calories). Then eat an additional 300 calories in the next two hours. Not only do you need to replace the fluids you lost, but you need to replace the carbohydrate depleted from your muscles.

workout diary

Goals:
_____
_____
_____

Dates:
_____

monday

STRETCHING ☐ DAILY RATING ☐

CARDIO EXERCISE	TIME/DISTANCE	NOTES
_____	_____	_____
_____	_____	_____
_____	_____	_____

STRENGTH TRAINING	WT.	SETS	REPS	NUTRITION NOTES
_____			
_____			
_____			
_____			
_____			
_____			
_____			
_____			
_____			
_____			

tuesday

STRETCHING ☐ DAILY RATING ☐

CARDIO EXERCISE	TIME/DISTANCE	NOTES
_____	_____	_____
_____	_____	_____
_____	_____	_____

STRENGTH TRAINING	WT.	SETS	REPS	NUTRITION NOTES
_____			
_____			
_____			
_____			
_____			
_____			
_____			
_____			
_____			
_____			

TRAINING TIP ■ *Doing zillions of sit-ups will not "whittle your middle," as the infomercials say. Abdominal exercises will strengthen and tone your ab muscles; to slim down, eat fewer calories and combine weight training with cardiovascular exercise.*

wednesday

STRETCHING ☐   DAILY RATING ☐

CARDIO EXERCISE _____   TIME/DISTANCE _____   NOTES _____

STRENGTH TRAINING _____   WT.   SETS   REPS

NUTRITION NOTES

thursday

STRETCHING ☐   DAILY RATING ☐

CARDIO EXERCISE _____   TIME/DISTANCE _____   NOTES _____

STRENGTH TRAINING _____   WT.   SETS   REPS

NUTRITION NOTES

> *"Focus on what is best for your training with your limited time available. Sometimes this means spending time with your family so you can keep things in balance."*
>
> *Scott Tinley, three-time Ironman World Series Triathlon Champion*

friday

STRETCHING ☐   DAILY RATING ☐

CARDIO EXERCISE	TIME/DISTANCE	NOTES

STRENGTH TRAINING	WT.	SETS	REPS

NUTRITION NOTES

saturday

STRETCHING ☐   DAILY RATING ☐

CARDIO EXERCISE	TIME/DISTANCE	NOTES

STRENGTH TRAINING	WT.	SETS	REPS

NUTRITION NOTES

sunday

STRETCHING ☐   DAILY RATING ☐

CARDIO EXERCISE   TIME/DISTANCE   NOTES

STRENGTH TRAINING   WT.   SETS   REPS

NUTRITION NOTES

weekly wrap-up

WEEKLY RATING ☐

GOALS: MET _____   EXCEEDED _____   MAYBE NEXT WEEK _____

CARDIO NOTES   STRENGTH NOTES

NUTRITION NOTES

TOTAL CARDIO SESSIONS ☐   TOTAL STRENGTH SESSIONS ☐   TOTAL STRETCHING SESSIONS ☐

Goals: _____

_____

_____

Dates: _____

monday

STRETCHING ☐   DAILY RATING ☐

CARDIO EXERCISE	TIME/DISTANCE	NOTES
_____	_____	_____
_____	_____	_____
_____	_____	_____

STRENGTH TRAINING	WT.	SETS	REPS
_____			
_____			
_____			
_____			
_____			
_____			
_____			
_____			
_____			
_____			

NUTRITION NOTES

tuesday

STRETCHING ☐   DAILY RATING ☐

CARDIO EXERCISE	TIME/DISTANCE	NOTES
_____	_____	_____
_____	_____	_____
_____	_____	_____

STRENGTH TRAINING	WT.	SETS	REPS
_____			
_____			
_____			
_____			
_____			
_____			
_____			
_____			
_____			

NUTRITION NOTES

RESEARCH REPORT ■ *Moderate exercise can boost your immune system. In a 15-week study, women who walked 45 minutes a day 5 days a week experienced fewer than half the sick days of women who didn't exercise. One caveat: over-training can suppress your immune system.*

wednesday

STRETCHING ☐　　DAILY RATING ☐

CARDIO EXERCISE　　TIME/DISTANCE　　NOTES

STRENGTH TRAINING　　WT.　SETS　REPS

NUTRITION NOTES

thursday

STRETCHING ☐　　DAILY RATING ☐

CARDIO EXERCISE　　TIME/DISTANCE　　NOTES

STRENGTH TRAINING　　WT.　SETS　REPS

NUTRITION NOTES

"My workout philosophy is, there's always another mountain. When I accomplish one goal, I want to take my training to a higher level."

Pamela McGee, professional basketball player, 1984 Olympic gold medalist

friday

STRETCHING [ ]   DAILY RATING [ ]

CARDIO EXERCISE	TIME/DISTANCE	NOTES

STRENGTH TRAINING	WT.	SETS	REPS

NUTRITION NOTES

saturday

STRETCHING [ ]   DAILY RATING [ ]

CARDIO EXERCISE	TIME/DISTANCE	NOTES

STRENGTH TRAINING	WT.	SETS	REPS

NUTRITION NOTES

sunday

STRETCHING ☐ DAILY RATING ☐

CARDIO EXERCISE | TIME/DISTANCE | NOTES

_____ | _____ | _____
_____ | _____ | _____
_____ | _____ | _____

STRENGTH TRAINING | WT. | SETS | REPS | **NUTRITION NOTES**

weekly wrap-up

WEEKLY RATING ☐

GOALS: MET _____   EXCEEDED _____   MAYBE NEXT WEEK _____

CARDIO NOTES | STRENGTH NOTES | **NUTRITION NOTES**

TOTAL CARDIO SESSIONS ☐   TOTAL STRENGTH SESSIONS ☐   TOTAL STRETCHING SESSIONS ☐

Goals: _____
_____
_____

Dates: _____

monday

STRETCHING ☐ DAILY RATING ☐

CARDIO EXERCISE	TIME/DISTANCE	NOTES
_____	_____	_____
_____	_____	_____
_____	_____	_____

STRENGTH TRAINING	WT.	SETS	REPS	NUTRITION NOTES
_____				
_____				
_____				
_____				
_____				
_____				
_____				
_____				
_____				
_____				

tuesday

STRETCHING ☐ DAILY RATING ☐

CARDIO EXERCISE	TIME/DISTANCE	NOTES
_____	_____	_____
_____	_____	_____
_____	_____	_____

STRENGTH TRAINING	WT.	SETS	REPS	NUTRITION NOTES
_____				
_____				
_____				
_____				
_____				
_____				
_____				
_____				
_____				
_____				

wednesday

STRETCHING ☐ DAILY RATING ☐

CARDIO EXERCISE	TIME/DISTANCE	NOTES

STRENGTH TRAINING	WT.	SETS	REPS

NUTRITION NOTES

thursday

STRETCHING ☐ DAILY RATING ☐

CARDIO EXERCISE	TIME/DISTANCE	NOTES

STRENGTH TRAINING	WT.	SETS	REPS

NUTRITION NOTES

"It's easy to get carried away while focused on a goal, so I use my log as insurance against overtraining. I track sick days, an indicator that I might be training too hard."

Tim Tweitmeyer, seven-time winner, Western States 100-mile Endurance Run

friday

STRETCHING ☐ DAILY RATING ☐

CARDIO EXERCISE	TIME/DISTANCE	NOTES

STRENGTH TRAINING	WT.	SETS	REPS	NUTRITION NOTES

saturday

STRETCHING ☐ DAILY RATING ☐

CARDIO EXERCISE	TIME/DISTANCE	NOTES

STRENGTH TRAINING	WT.	SETS	REPS	NUTRITION NOTES

sunday

STRETCHING ☐   DAILY RATING ☐

CARDIO EXERCISE _____   TIME/DISTANCE _____   NOTES _____

STRENGTH TRAINING _____   WT.   SETS   REPS

NUTRITION NOTES

weekly wrap-up

WEEKLY RATING ☐

GOALS: MET _____   EXCEEDED _____   MAYBE NEXT WEEK _____

CARDIO NOTES _____   STRENGTH NOTES _____

NUTRITION NOTES

TOTAL CARDIO SESSIONS ☐   TOTAL STRENGTH SESSIONS ☐   TOTAL STRETCHING SESSIONS ☐

4

Goals:

Dates:

monday

STRETCHING ☐   DAILY RATING ☐

CARDIO EXERCISE	TIME/DISTANCE	NOTES

STRENGTH TRAINING	WT.	SETS	REPS	NUTRITION NOTES

tuesday

STRETCHING ☐   DAILY RATING ☐

CARDIO EXERCISE	TIME/DISTANCE	NOTES

STRENGTH TRAINING	WT.	SETS	REPS	NUTRITION NOTES

RESEARCH REPORT ■ *Exercise can help you sleep better. In a 12-week study, subjects on an aerobic and strength-training program reported falling asleep faster, sleeping longer, and waking up less frequently than before they started exercising.*

wednesday

STRETCHING ☐   DAILY RATING ☐

CARDIO EXERCISE	TIME/DISTANCE	NOTES

STRENGTH TRAINING	WT.	SETS	REPS	NUTRITION NOTES

thursday

STRETCHING ☐   DAILY RATING ☐

CARDIO EXERCISE	TIME/DISTANCE	NOTES

STRENGTH TRAINING	WT.	SETS	REPS	NUTRITION NOTES

> **"When you look back at your log and see all the work you've put in, it's definitely a confidence booster."**
>
> *Amy Rudolph, American record-holder, 5,000-meter run*

friday

STRETCHING ☐ DAILY RATING ☐

CARDIO EXERCISE	TIME/DISTANCE	NOTES

STRENGTH TRAINING	WT.	SETS	REPS	NUTRITION NOTES

saturday

STRETCHING ☐ DAILY RATING ☐

CARDIO EXERCISE	TIME/DISTANCE	NOTES

STRENGTH TRAINING	WT.	SETS	REPS	NUTRITION NOTES

SPORTSPEAK ■ *Roll up the windows: When a skier takes a jump off-balance and swings his or her arms in circles. Usage: "That dude can't jump; he's always rolling up the windows."*

sunday

STRETCHING ☐   DAILY RATING ☐

CARDIO EXERCISE	TIME/DISTANCE	NOTES

STRENGTH TRAINING	WT.	SETS	REPS	NUTRITION NOTES

weekly wrap-up

WEEKLY RATING ☐

GOALS: MET _____   EXCEEDED _____   MAYBE NEXT WEEK _____

CARDIO NOTES	STRENGTH NOTES	NUTRITION NOTES

TOTAL CARDIO SESSIONS ☐

TOTAL STRENGTH SESSIONS ☐

TOTAL STRETCHING SESSIONS ☐

Goals:

Dates:

monday

STRETCHING ☐   DAILY RATING ☐

CARDIO EXERCISE	TIME/DISTANCE	NOTES

STRENGTH TRAINING	WT.	SETS	REPS

NUTRITION NOTES

tuesday

STRETCHING ☐   DAILY RATING ☐

CARDIO EXERCISE	TIME/DISTANCE	NOTES

STRENGTH TRAINING	WT.	SETS	REPS

NUTRITION NOTES

TRAINING TIP ■ *Drinking 8 glasses of water a day isn't enough for most active people. The simplest way to tell if you're well hydrated is to monitor your urine. If it's dark and scanty instead of clear and plentiful, you need to drink more.*

wednesday

STRETCHING ☐   DAILY RATING ☐

CARDIO EXERCISE	TIME/DISTANCE	NOTES

STRENGTH TRAINING	WT.	SETS	REPS	NUTRITION NOTES

thursday

STRETCHING ☐   DAILY RATING ☐

CARDIO EXERCISE	TIME/DISTANCE	NOTES

STRENGTH TRAINING	WT.	SETS	REPS	NUTRITION NOTES

> *"It's important to keep a log even in the off season or through injuries. It helps me keep track of the ebb and flow of my body's natural rhythms, which helps me plan my seasons for the future."*
>
> *Shari Kain, National Mountain Bike Triathlon Champion, Tour de France veteran*

friday

STRETCHING ☐　　DAILY RATING ☐

CARDIO EXERCISE	TIME/DISTANCE	NOTES

STRENGTH TRAINING	WT.	SETS	REPS	NUTRITION NOTES

saturday

STRETCHING ☐　　DAILY RATING ☐

CARDIO EXERCISE	TIME/DISTANCE	NOTES

STRENGTH TRAINING	WT.	SETS	REPS	NUTRITION NOTES

sunday

STRETCHING ☐   DAILY RATING ☐

CARDIO EXERCISE _____   TIME/DISTANCE _____   NOTES _____

_____   _____   _____
_____   _____   _____
_____   _____   _____

STRENGTH TRAINING _____   WT.   SETS   REPS

NUTRITION NOTES

weekly wrap-up

WEEKLY RATING ☐

GOALS: MET _____   EXCEEDED _____   MAYBE NEXT WEEK _____

CARDIO NOTES _____   STRENGTH NOTES _____

NUTRITION NOTES

TOTAL CARDIO SESSIONS ☐   TOTAL STRENGTH SESSIONS ☐   TOTAL STRETCHING SESSIONS ☐

Goals: _____
_____
_____

Dates: _____

monday

STRETCHING ☐   DAILY RATING ☐

CARDIO EXERCISE	TIME/DISTANCE	NOTES
_____	_____	_____
_____	_____	_____
_____	_____	_____

STRENGTH TRAINING	WT.	SETS	REPS	NUTRITION NOTES
_____				
_____				
_____				
_____				
_____				
_____				
_____				
_____				
_____				
_____				

tuesday

STRETCHING ☐   DAILY RATING ☐

CARDIO EXERCISE	TIME/DISTANCE	NOTES
_____	_____	_____
_____	_____	_____
_____	_____	_____

STRENGTH TRAINING	WT.	SETS	REPS	NUTRITION NOTES
_____				
_____				
_____				
_____				
_____				
_____				
_____				
_____				

RESEARCH REPORT ■ *It's never too late to benefit from lifting weights. After an 8-week strength-training program, seniors aged 86 to 96 increased their strength, walking speed, and balance dramatically. Two men in the study even discarded their canes.*

wednesday

STRETCHING ☐   DAILY RATING ☐

CARDIO EXERCISE   TIME/DISTANCE   NOTES

STRENGTH TRAINING   WT.   SETS   REPS

NUTRITION NOTES

thursday

STRETCHING ☐   DAILY RATING ☐

CARDIO EXERCISE   TIME/DISTANCE   NOTES

STRENGTH TRAINING   WT.   SETS   REPS

NUTRITION NOTES

> *"You'll only reach your competitive potential and achieve your fitness goals when you can exercise for pure enjoyment, regardless of your times or mileage or the demands of your ego."*
>
> Brad Kearns, world-class professional triathlete

friday

STRETCHING ☐ DAILY RATING ☐

CARDIO EXERCISE	TIME/DISTANCE	NOTES
_____	_____	_____
_____	_____	_____
_____	_____	_____
_____	_____	_____

STRENGTH TRAINING	WT.	SETS	REPS
_____			
_____			
_____			
_____			
_____			
_____			
_____			
_____			
_____			
_____			

NUTRITION NOTES

saturday

STRETCHING ☐ DAILY RATING ☐

CARDIO EXERCISE	TIME/DISTANCE	NOTES
_____	_____	_____
_____	_____	_____
_____	_____	_____
_____	_____	_____

STRENGTH TRAINING	WT.	SETS	REPS
_____			
_____			
_____			
_____			
_____			
_____			
_____			
_____			
_____			
_____			

NUTRITION NOTES

sunday

STRETCHING ☐   DAILY RATING ☐

CARDIO EXERCISE   TIME/DISTANCE   NOTES

STRENGTH TRAINING   WT.   SETS   REPS

NUTRITION NOTES

weekly wrap-up

WEEKLY RATING ☐

GOALS: MET _____   EXCEEDED _____   MAYBE NEXT WEEK _____

CARDIO NOTES   STRENGTH NOTES

NUTRITION NOTES

TOTAL CARDIO SESSIONS ☐   TOTAL STRENGTH SESSIONS ☐   TOTAL STRETCHING SESSIONS ☐

Goals:

Dates:

monday

STRETCHING ☐ DAILY RATING ☐

CARDIO EXERCISE   TIME/DISTANCE   NOTES

STRENGTH TRAINING   WT.   SETS   REPS

NUTRITION NOTES

tuesday

STRETCHING ☐ DAILY RATING ☐

CARDIO EXERCISE   TIME/DISTANCE   NOTES

STRENGTH TRAINING   WT.   SETS   REPS

NUTRITION NOTES

TRAINING TIP ■ *If one side of your body is more than 10 percent stronger than the other, you may not perform to your potential and may end up with injuries. To balance out your muscle strength, include dumbbells in your strength program; they'll force each side to pull its own weight.*

wednesday

STRETCHING ☐   DAILY RATING ☐

CARDIO EXERCISE	TIME/DISTANCE	NOTES

STRENGTH TRAINING	WT.	SETS	REPS	NUTRITION NOTES

thursday

STRETCHING ☐   DAILY RATING ☐

CARDIO EXERCISE	TIME/DISTANCE	NOTES

STRENGTH TRAINING	WT.	SETS	REPS	NUTRITION NOTES

"I'm motivated to achieve my goals by the challenge of proving people wrong. There is nothing like the feeling of doing something that others thought you could never do."

Alexi Lalas, 1992 and 1996 Olympic soccer team member

friday.

STRETCHING ☐   DAILY RATING ☐

CARDIO EXERCISE	TIME/DISTANCE	NOTES

STRENGTH TRAINING	WT.	SETS	REPS	NUTRITION NOTES

saturday

STRETCHING ☐   DAILY RATING ☐

CARDIO EXERCISE	TIME/DISTANCE	NOTES

STRENGTH TRAINING	WT.	SETS	REPS	NUTRITION NOTES

sunday

STRETCHING ☐ DAILY RATING ☐

CARDIO EXERCISE	TIME/DISTANCE	NOTES

STRENGTH TRAINING	WT.	SETS	REPS	NUTRITION NOTES

weekly wrap-up

WEEKLY RATING ☐

GOALS: MET _____ EXCEEDED _____ MAYBE NEXT WEEK _____

CARDIO NOTES	STRENGTH NOTES	NUTRITION NOTES

TOTAL CARDIO SESSIONS ☐   TOTAL STRENGTH SESSIONS ☐   TOTAL STRETCHING SESSIONS ☐

Goals: _____
_____
_____

Dates: _____

monday

STRETCHING ☐   DAILY RATING ☐

CARDIO EXERCISE	TIME/DISTANCE	NOTES
_____	_____	_____
_____	_____	_____
_____	_____	_____

STRENGTH TRAINING	WT.	SETS	REPS	NUTRITION NOTES
_____				
_____				
_____				
_____				
_____				
_____				
_____				
_____				
_____				
_____				

tuesday

STRETCHING ☐   DAILY RATING ☐

CARDIO EXERCISE	TIME/DISTANCE	NOTES
_____	_____	_____
_____	_____	_____
_____	_____	_____

STRENGTH TRAINING	WT.	SETS	REPS	NUTRITION NOTES
_____				
_____				
_____				
_____				
_____				
_____				
_____				
_____				
_____				
_____				

RESEARCH REPORT ■ *To get fit and lose weight, you don't need to exercise in long bouts. In a 10-week study, women who walked three times a day for 10 minutes lost as much fat and gained as much fitness as those who exercised in one 30-minute session.*

wednesday

STRETCHING ☐   DAILY RATING ☐

CARDIO EXERCISE	TIME/DISTANCE	NOTES
_____	_____	_____
_____	_____	_____
_____	_____	_____

STRENGTH TRAINING	WT.	SETS	REPS	NUTRITION NOTES
_____				
_____				
_____				
_____				
_____				
_____				
_____				
_____				
_____				
_____				

thursday

STRETCHING ☐   DAILY RATING ☐

CARDIO EXERCISE	TIME/DISTANCE	NOTES
_____	_____	_____
_____	_____	_____
_____	_____	_____

STRENGTH TRAINING	WT.	SETS	REPS	NUTRITION NOTES
_____				
_____				
_____				
_____				
_____				
_____				
_____				
_____				
_____				
_____				

"When my teammates are cheering me on, I don't want to let them down or let myself down. You might as well suck it up and do it. You feel ten times better when you're done."

Sally Oates, 2000 Olympic weightlifting team member

friday

STRETCHING ☐ DAILY RATING ☐

CARDIO EXERCISE	TIME/DISTANCE	NOTES

STRENGTH TRAINING	WT.	SETS	REPS

NUTRITION NOTES

saturday

STRETCHING ☐ DAILY RATING ☐

CARDIO EXERCISE	TIME/DISTANCE	NOTES

STRENGTH TRAINING	WT.	SETS	REPS

NUTRITION NOTES

sunday

STRETCHING ☐   DAILY RATING ☐

CARDIO EXERCISE _____   TIME/DISTANCE _____   NOTES _____

_____   _____   _____
_____   _____   _____
_____   _____   _____

STRENGTH TRAINING   WT.   SETS   REPS   NUTRITION NOTES

_____
_____
_____
_____
_____
_____
_____
_____
_____
_____
_____

weekly wrap-up

WEEKLY RATING ☐

GOALS: MET _____   EXCEEDED _____   MAYBE NEXT WEEK _____

CARDIO NOTES   STRENGTH NOTES   NUTRITION NOTES

_____   _____
_____   _____
_____   _____
_____   _____
_____   _____
_____   _____
_____   _____
_____   _____
_____   _____

TOTAL CARDIO SESSIONS ☐   TOTAL STRENGTH SESSIONS ☐   TOTAL STRETCHING SESSIONS ☐

Goals:

Dates:

monday

STRETCHING ☐   DAILY RATING ☐

CARDIO EXERCISE	TIME/DISTANCE	NOTES

STRENGTH TRAINING	WT.	SETS	REPS	NUTRITION NOTES

tuesday

STRETCHING ☐   DAILY RATING ☐

CARDIO EXERCISE	TIME/DISTANCE	NOTES

STRENGTH TRAINING	WT.	SETS	REPS	NUTRITION NOTES

TRAINING TIP ◼ *When you start lifting weights, don't be alarmed if you gain weight. Muscle takes up less room than fat but weighs more per square inch. So, while the needle on the scale may inch upward, your clothing may get looser.*

wednesday

STRETCHING ☐   DAILY RATING ☐

CARDIO EXERCISE	TIME/DISTANCE	NOTES

STRENGTH TRAINING	WT.	SETS	REPS	NUTRITION NOTES

thursday

STRETCHING ☐   DAILY RATING ☐

CARDIO EXERCISE	TIME/DISTANCE	NOTES

STRENGTH TRAINING	WT.	SETS	REPS	NUTRITION NOTES

> *"I've found that a goal too closely held can take on a life of its own. Now is all there is, so handle what life is giving you now."*
>
> Paula Newby-Fraser, seven-time winner, Hawaii Ironman Triathlon

friday

STRETCHING ☐ DAILY RATING ☐

CARDIO EXERCISE	TIME/DISTANCE	NOTES

STRENGTH TRAINING	WT.	SETS	REPS

NUTRITION NOTES

saturday

STRETCHING ☐ DAILY RATING ☐

CARDIO EXERCISE	TIME/DISTANCE	NOTES

STRENGTH TRAINING	WT.	SETS	REPS

NUTRITION NOTES

SPORTSPEAK ■ *Hip check (n.): When a skier lands after a jump and bounces off his or her hip. Usage: "She almost stuck her landing, but that hip check looked painful."*

sunday

STRETCHING ☐ DAILY RATING ☐

CARDIO EXERCISE   TIME/DISTANCE   NOTES

STRENGTH TRAINING   WT.   SETS   REPS

NUTRITION NOTES

weekly wrap-up

WEEKLY RATING ☐

GOALS: MET _____   EXCEEDED _____   MAYBE NEXT WEEK _____

CARDIO NOTES   STRENGTH NOTES

NUTRITION NOTES

TOTAL CARDIO SESSIONS ☐   TOTAL STRENGTH SESSIONS ☐   TOTAL STRETCHING SESSIONS ☐

Goals: _____

Dates: _____

monday

STRETCHING ☐   DAILY RATING ☐

CARDIO EXERCISE	TIME/DISTANCE	NOTES
_____	_____	_____
_____	_____	_____
_____	_____	_____

STRENGTH TRAINING	WT.	SETS	REPS	NUTRITION NOTES
_____				
_____				
_____				
_____				
_____				
_____				
_____				
_____				
_____				
_____				
_____				

tuesday

STRETCHING ☐   DAILY RATING ☐

CARDIO EXERCISE	TIME/DISTANCE	NOTES
_____	_____	_____
_____	_____	_____
_____	_____	_____

STRENGTH TRAINING	WT.	SETS	REPS	NUTRITION NOTES
_____				
_____				
_____				
_____				
_____				
_____				
_____				
_____				
_____				
_____				

RESEARCH REPORT ■ *Fitness matters more than thinness. In one study, unfit thin men died prematurely three times more often than overweight men who exercised three to five times a week.*

wednesday

STRETCHING ☐ DAILY RATING ☐

CARDIO EXERCISE	TIME/DISTANCE	NOTES

STRENGTH TRAINING	WT.	SETS	REPS

NUTRITION NOTES

thursday

STRETCHING ☐ DAILY RATING ☐

CARDIO EXERCISE	TIME/DISTANCE	NOTES

STRENGTH TRAINING	WT.	SETS	REPS

NUTRITION NOTES

"I set 'wish goals,' like an Olympic gold medal, and performance goals, like finishing in the top ten in a particular race. To reach these, I set training goals. It's a step-by-step process."

Kyle Rasmussen, 1998 Olympic downhill skier

friday

STRETCHING ☐   DAILY RATING ☐

CARDIO EXERCISE	TIME/DISTANCE	NOTES

STRENGTH TRAINING	WT.	SETS	REPS

NUTRITION NOTES

saturday

STRETCHING ☐   DAILY RATING ☐

CARDIO EXERCISE	TIME/DISTANCE	NOTES

STRENGTH TRAINING	WT.	SETS	REPS

NUTRITION NOTES

sunday

STRETCHING ☐   DAILY RATING ☐

CARDIO EXERCISE

TIME/DISTANCE

NOTES

STRENGTH TRAINING   WT.   SETS   REPS   **NUTRITION NOTES**

weekly wrap-up

WEEKLY RATING ☐

GOALS: MET _____   EXCEEDED _____   MAYBE NEXT WEEK _____

CARDIO NOTES

STRENGTH NOTES

NUTRITION NOTES

TOTAL CARDIO SESSIONS ☐

TOTAL STRENGTH SESSIONS ☐

TOTAL STRETCHING SESSIONS ☐

11

Goals: _____

_____

_____

Dates: _____

monday

STRETCHING ☐   DAILY RATING ☐

CARDIO EXERCISE	TIME/DISTANCE	NOTES
_____	_____	_____
_____	_____	_____
_____	_____	_____

STRENGTH TRAINING	WT.	SETS	REPS	NUTRITION NOTES
_____				
_____				
_____				
_____				
_____				
_____				
_____				
_____				
_____				
_____				

tuesday

STRETCHING ☐   DAILY RATING ☐

CARDIO EXERCISE	TIME/DISTANCE	NOTES
_____	_____	_____
_____	_____	_____
_____	_____	_____

STRENGTH TRAINING	WT.	SETS	REPS	NUTRITION NOTES
_____				
_____				
_____				
_____				
_____				
_____				
_____				
_____				
_____				

TRAINING TIP ■ *Conventional wisdom has it that sports drinks are help-ful only if you exercise continuously for an hour or more. But new studies suggest that sports drinks can improve performance for stop-and-go sports and for workouts last-ing less than an hour.*

wednesday

STRETCHING ☐ DAILY RATING ☐

CARDIO EXERCISE	TIME/DISTANCE	NOTES
_____	_____	_____
_____	_____	_____
_____	_____	_____

STRENGTH TRAINING	WT.	SETS	REPS	NUTRITION NOTES
_____				
_____				
_____				
_____				
_____				
_____				
_____				
_____				
_____				
_____				

thursday

STRETCHING ☐ DAILY RATING ☐

CARDIO EXERCISE	TIME/DISTANCE	NOTES
_____	_____	_____
_____	_____	_____
_____	_____	_____

STRENGTH TRAINING	WT.	SETS	REPS	NUTRITION NOTES
_____				
_____				
_____				
_____				
_____				
_____				
_____				
_____				

"I've kept a training log for the last twenty-three years. There is no better reference tool to see how I successfully prepare for a peak performance."

Greg Demgen, ten-year National Cycling Team member

friday

STRETCHING ☐   DAILY RATING ☐

CARDIO EXERCISE	TIME/DISTANCE	NOTES

STRENGTH TRAINING	WT.	SETS	REPS	NUTRITION NOTES

saturday

STRETCHING ☐   DAILY RATING ☐

CARDIO EXERCISE	TIME/DISTANCE	NOTES

STRENGTH TRAINING	WT.	SETS	REPS	NUTRITION NOTES

sunday

STRETCHING ☐ DAILY RATING ☐

CARDIO EXERCISE _____ TIME/DISTANCE _____ NOTES _____

STRENGTH TRAINING _____ WT. SETS REPS

NUTRITION NOTES

weekly wrap-up

WEEKLY RATING ☐

GOALS: MET _____ EXCEEDED _____ MAYBE NEXT WEEK _____

CARDIO NOTES _____ STRENGTH NOTES _____

NUTRITION NOTES

TOTAL CARDIO SESSIONS ☐

TOTAL STRENGTH SESSIONS ☐

TOTAL STRETCHING SESSIONS ☐

Goals: _____

_____

_____

Dates: _____

monday

STRETCHING ☐   DAILY RATING ☐

CARDIO EXERCISE	TIME/DISTANCE	NOTES
_____	_____	_____
_____	_____	_____
_____	_____	_____

STRENGTH TRAINING	WT.	SETS	REPS
_____			
_____			
_____			
_____			
_____			
_____			
_____			
_____			
_____			
_____			
_____			

NUTRITION NOTES

tuesday

STRETCHING ☐   DAILY RATING ☐

CARDIO EXERCISE	TIME/DISTANCE	NOTES
_____	_____	_____
_____	_____	_____
_____	_____	_____

STRENGTH TRAINING	WT.	SETS	REPS
_____			
_____			
_____			
_____			
_____			
_____			
_____			
_____			
_____			

NUTRITION NOTES

RESEARCH REPORT ▮ *Exercise is the key to keeping off weight. In one study, dieters lost twice as much weight as exercisers who did not restrict their food intake. But after one year, the dieters gained all their weight back and more; the exercisers maintained their average six-pound weight loss.*

wednesday

STRETCHING ☐   DAILY RATING ☐

CARDIO EXERCISE _____   TIME/DISTANCE _____   NOTES _____

STRENGTH TRAINING _____   WT.   SETS   REPS

NUTRITION NOTES

thursday

STRETCHING ☐   DAILY RATING ☐

CARDIO EXERCISE _____   TIME/DISTANCE _____   NOTES _____

STRENGTH TRAINING _____   WT.   SETS   REPS

NUTRITION NOTES

"Seeing yourself improve is a big motivator. That's what keeps me going—improving and having people cheer for you. That really pumps me up." Pete Kelley, weightlifter, 1996 Olympian

friday

STRETCHING ☐ DAILY RATING ☐

CARDIO EXERCISE	TIME/DISTANCE	NOTES

STRENGTH TRAINING	WT.	SETS	REPS

NUTRITION NOTES

saturday

STRETCHING ☐ DAILY RATING ☐

CARDIO EXERCISE	TIME/DISTANCE	NOTES

STRENGTH TRAINING	WT.	SETS	REPS

NUTRITION NOTES

sunday

STRETCHING ☐   DAILY RATING ☐

CARDIO EXERCISE   TIME/DISTANCE   NOTES

_____   _____   _____
_____   _____   _____
_____   _____   _____
_____   _____   _____

STRENGTH TRAINING   WT.   SETS   REPS

NUTRITION NOTES

weekly wrap-up

WEEKLY RATING ☐

GOALS: MET _____   EXCEEDED _____   MAYBE NEXT WEEK _____

CARDIO NOTES   STRENGTH NOTES   **NUTRITION NOTES**

TOTAL CARDIO SESSIONS ☐   TOTAL STRENGTH SESSIONS ☐   TOTAL STRETCHING SESSIONS ☐

13

Goals: _____

_____

_____

Dates: _____

monday

STRETCHING ☐ DAILY RATING ☐

CARDIO EXERCISE	TIME/DISTANCE	NOTES

STRENGTH TRAINING	WT.	SETS	REPS

NUTRITION NOTES

tuesday

STRETCHING ☐ DAILY RATING ☐

CARDIO EXERCISE	TIME/DISTANCE	NOTES

STRENGTH TRAINING	WT.	SETS	REPS

NUTRITION NOTES

TRAINING TIP ■ *Beware of fitness programs advertised as being better than anything in existence. There's no single regimen that works best for everyone. Experiment with a variety of plans and don't get sucked in by sensational magazine headlines or diet claims.*

wednesday

STRETCHING ☐ DAILY RATING ☐

CARDIO EXERCISE	TIME/DISTANCE	NOTES

STRENGTH TRAINING	WT.	SETS	REPS	NUTRITION NOTES

thursday

STRETCHING ☐ DAILY RATING ☐

CARDIO EXERCISE	TIME/DISTANCE	NOTES

STRENGTH TRAINING	WT.	SETS	REPS	NUTRITION NOTES

"When I'm feeling lazy, I just remind myself how good I feel after I work out." *Sandy Dukat, disabled swimmer and downhill ski racer*

friday

STRETCHING ☐   DAILY RATING ☐

CARDIO EXERCISE	TIME/DISTANCE	NOTES

STRENGTH TRAINING	WT.	SETS	REPS	NUTRITION NOTES

saturday

STRETCHING ☐   DAILY RATING ☐

CARDIO EXERCISE	TIME/DISTANCE	NOTES

STRENGTH TRAINING	WT.	SETS	REPS	NUTRITION NOTES

SPORTSPEAK ■ *Flash (v.): To climb a rock on the first try without falling. Usage: "She's the only one who has flashed this climb."*

sunday

STRETCHING ☐

DAILY RATING ☐

CARDIO EXERCISE _____   TIME/DISTANCE _____   NOTES _____

_____   _____   _____
_____   _____   _____
_____   _____   _____

STRENGTH TRAINING _____

WT.	SETS	REPS

NUTRITION NOTES

weekly wrap-up

WEEKLY RATING ☐

GOALS: MET _____   EXCEEDED _____   MAYBE NEXT WEEK _____

CARDIO NOTES _____   STRENGTH NOTES _____

_____   _____
_____   _____
_____   _____
_____   _____
_____   _____
_____   _____
_____   _____
_____   _____

NUTRITION NOTES

TOTAL CARDIO SESSIONS ☐   TOTAL STRENGTH SESSIONS ☐   TOTAL STRETCHING SESSIONS ☐

Goals: _____
_____
_____

Dates: _____

monday

STRETCHING ☐ DAILY RATING ☐

CARDIO EXERCISE	TIME/DISTANCE	NOTES
_____	_____	_____
_____	_____	_____
_____	_____	_____

STRENGTH TRAINING	WT.	SETS	REPS
_____			
_____			
_____			
_____			
_____			
_____			
_____			
_____			
_____			
_____			

NUTRITION NOTES

tuesday

STRETCHING ☐ DAILY RATING ☐

CARDIO EXERCISE	TIME/DISTANCE	NOTES
_____	_____	_____
_____	_____	_____
_____	_____	_____

STRENGTH TRAINING	WT.	SETS	REPS
_____			
_____			
_____			
_____			
_____			
_____			
_____			
_____			
_____			

NUTRITION NOTES

RESEARCH REPORT ■ *Working out with a partner will help you stick with your program. In one study, married couples who exercised together had a 40 percent higher attendance rate at an exercise class than married people who went to the class separately.*

wednesday

STRETCHING ☐   DAILY RATING ☐

CARDIO EXERCISE	TIME/DISTANCE	NOTES

STRENGTH TRAINING	WT.	SETS	REPS

NUTRITION NOTES

thursday

STRETCHING ☐   DAILY RATING ☐

CARDIO EXERCISE	TIME/DISTANCE	NOTES

STRENGTH TRAINING	WT.	SETS	REPS

NUTRITION NOTES

"I try not to let off-days get to me. If I'm not able to accomplish what I want on a certain day, I relax and visualize what needs to be done."

Tim McRae, weightlifter, 1996 Olympian

friday

STRETCHING ☐   DAILY RATING ☐

CARDIO EXERCISE	TIME/DISTANCE	NOTES
_____	_____	_____
_____	_____	_____
_____	_____	_____

STRENGTH TRAINING	WT.	SETS	REPS	NUTRITION NOTES
_____				
_____				
_____				
_____				
_____				
_____				
_____				
_____				
_____				
_____				

saturday

STRETCHING ☐   DAILY RATING ☐

CARDIO EXERCISE	TIME/DISTANCE	NOTES
_____	_____	_____
_____	_____	_____
_____	_____	_____

STRENGTH TRAINING	WT.	SETS	REPS	NUTRITION NOTES
_____				
_____				
_____				
_____				
_____				
_____				
_____				
_____				
_____				
_____				

SPORTSPEAK ■ *Head dab (n.): A unintentional maneuver pitting a mountain biker's head against a rock, tree, or other inanimate object. Chi chi (n.): First aid. Usage: "That guy just did a major head dab. Maybe he needs some chi chi."*

sunday

STRETCHING ☐   DAILY RATING ☐

CARDIO EXERCISE   TIME/DISTANCE   NOTES

STRENGTH TRAINING   WT.   SETS   REPS

NUTRITION NOTES

weekly wrap-up

WEEKLY RATING ☐

GOALS: MET _____   EXCEEDED _____   MAYBE NEXT WEEK _____

CARDIO NOTES   STRENGTH NOTES

NUTRITION NOTES

TOTAL CARDIO SESSIONS ☐   TOTAL STRENGTH SESSIONS ☐   TOTAL STRETCHING SESSIONS ☐

Goals: _____

_____

_____

Dates: _____

monday

STRETCHING ☐ DAILY RATING ☐

CARDIO EXERCISE	TIME/DISTANCE	NOTES
_____	_____	_____
_____	_____	_____
_____	_____	_____
_____	_____	_____

STRENGTH TRAINING	WT.	SETS	REPS
_____			
_____			
_____			
_____			
_____			
_____			
_____			
_____			
_____			
_____			

NUTRITION NOTES

tuesday

STRETCHING ☐ DAILY RATING ☐

CARDIO EXERCISE	TIME/DISTANCE	NOTES
_____	_____	_____
_____	_____	_____
_____	_____	_____

STRENGTH TRAINING	WT.	SETS	REPS
_____			
_____			
_____			
_____			
_____			
_____			
_____			
_____			
_____			

NUTRITION NOTES

TRAINING TIP ■ *Bored with stairclimbing machines? Try climbing real steps. It's a tougher workout; you can't cheat by hugging the console or by taking shorter steps when you get tired.*

wednesday

STRETCHING ☐   DAILY RATING ☐

CARDIO EXERCISE	TIME/DISTANCE	NOTES

STRENGTH TRAINING	WT.	SETS	REPS	NUTRITION NOTES

thursday

STRETCHING ☐   DAILY RATING ☐

CARDIO EXERCISE	TIME/DISTANCE	NOTES

STRENGTH TRAINING	WT.	SETS	REPS	NUTRITION NOTES

> *"Quality rest is just as important as quality training. After training hard for six days, how can you expect to recover in one day?"*
>
> *Michellie Jones, two-time Triathlon World Series champion*

friday

STRETCHING ☐   DAILY RATING ☐

CARDIO EXERCISE	TIME/DISTANCE	NOTES

STRENGTH TRAINING	WT.	SETS	REPS	NUTRITION NOTES

saturday

STRETCHING ☐   DAILY RATING ☐

CARDIO EXERCISE	TIME/DISTANCE	NOTES

STRENGTH TRAINING	WT.	SETS	REPS	NUTRITION NOTES

sunday

STRETCHING ☐   DAILY RATING ☐

CARDIO EXERCISE   TIME/DISTANCE   NOTES

_____   _____   _____
_____   _____   _____
_____   _____   _____
_____   _____   _____

STRENGTH TRAINING	WT.	SETS	REPS	**NUTRITION NOTES**
_____				
_____				
_____				
_____				
_____				
_____				
_____				
_____				
_____				
_____				

weekly wrap-up

WEEKLY RATING ☐

GOALS: MET _____   EXCEEDED _____   MAYBE NEXT WEEK _____

CARDIO NOTES   STRENGTH NOTES   **NUTRITION NOTES**

_____   _____
_____   _____
_____   _____
_____   _____
_____   _____
_____   _____
_____   _____
_____   _____
_____   _____
_____   _____
_____   _____

TOTAL CARDIO SESSIONS ☐   TOTAL STRENGTH SESSIONS ☐   TOTAL STRETCHING SESSIONS ☐

Goals: _____

_____

Dates: _____

monday

STRETCHING ☐ DAILY RATING ☐

CARDIO EXERCISE	TIME/DISTANCE	NOTES
_____	_____	_____
_____	_____	_____
_____	_____	_____

STRENGTH TRAINING	WT.	SETS	REPS	NUTRITION NOTES
_____				
_____				
_____				
_____				
_____				
_____				
_____				
_____				
_____				
_____				

tuesday

STRETCHING ☐ DAILY RATING ☐

CARDIO EXERCISE	TIME/DISTANCE	NOTES
_____	_____	_____
_____	_____	_____
_____	_____	_____

STRENGTH TRAINING	WT.	SETS	REPS	NUTRITION NOTES
_____				
_____				
_____				
_____				
_____				
_____				
_____				
_____				
_____				
_____				

RESEARCH REPORT ■ *Walking can save lives. In a 12-year study, retired, nonsmoking men who walked at least 2 miles a day had only about half as many deaths as those who walked less than 1 mile a day.*

wednesday

STRETCHING ☐   DAILY RATING ☐

CARDIO EXERCISE	TIME/DISTANCE	NOTES

STRENGTH TRAINING	WT.	SETS	REPS	NUTRITION NOTES

thursday

STRETCHING ☐   DAILY RATING ☐

CARDIO EXERCISE	TIME/DISTANCE	NOTES

STRENGTH TRAINING	WT.	SETS	REPS	NUTRITION NOTES

"It helps to be flexible and spontaneous. I make sure I stay on track with my goal in sight, but I'm able to adjust my schedule day-to-day."

Lynn Hill, world-class rock climber

friday

STRETCHING ☐   DAILY RATING ☐

CARDIO EXERCISE	TIME/DISTANCE	NOTES

STRENGTH TRAINING	WT.	SETS	REPS

NUTRITION NOTES

saturday

STRETCHING ☐   DAILY RATING ☐

CARDIO EXERCISE	TIME/DISTANCE	NOTES

STRENGTH TRAINING	WT.	SETS	REPS

NUTRITION NOTES

sunday

STRETCHING ☐ DAILY RATING ☐

CARDIO EXERCISE _____ TIME/DISTANCE _____ NOTES _____

_____ _____ _____
_____ _____ _____
_____ _____ _____

STRENGTH TRAINING _____ WT. SETS REPS

NUTRITION NOTES

weekly wrap-up

WEEKLY RATING ☐

GOALS: MET _____ EXCEEDED _____ MAYBE NEXT WEEK _____

CARDIO NOTES _____ STRENGTH NOTES _____

NUTRITION NOTES

TOTAL CARDIO SESSIONS ☐   TOTAL STRENGTH SESSIONS ☐   TOTAL STRETCHING SESSIONS ☐

17

Goals:

Dates:

monday

STRETCHING ☐   DAILY RATING ☐

CARDIO EXERCISE	TIME/DISTANCE	NOTES

STRENGTH TRAINING	WT.	SETS	REPS

NUTRITION NOTES

tuesday

STRETCHING ☐   DAILY RATING ☐

CARDIO EXERCISE	TIME/DISTANCE	NOTES

STRENGTH TRAINING	WT.	SETS	REPS

NUTRITION NOTES

TRAINING TIP ■ *It's a myth that low-intensity exercise burns more fat than high-intensity exercise. What matters for weight loss is how many total calories you burn. High-intensity exercise burns more calories per minute, but the advantage of exercising at an easy pace is that you can sustain it longer.*

wednesday

STRETCHING ☐   DAILY RATING ☐

CARDIO EXERCISE _____   TIME/DISTANCE _____   NOTES _____

_____   _____   _____
_____   _____   _____
_____   _____   _____

STRENGTH TRAINING _____   WT.   SETS   REPS   **NUTRITION NOTES**

_____
_____
_____
_____
_____
_____
_____
_____
_____

thursday

STRETCHING ☐   DAILY RATING ☐

CARDIO EXERCISE _____   TIME/DISTANCE _____   NOTES _____

_____   _____   _____
_____   _____   _____

STRENGTH TRAINING _____   WT.   SETS   REPS   **NUTRITION NOTES**

_____
_____
_____
_____
_____
_____
_____
_____
_____

"When I was training for the Olympics, I'd check my workout journal to make sure I was improving. I figured that way I was held responsible for what I was doing."

Kurt Grote, swimmer, 1996 Olympian

friday

STRETCHING ☐　DAILY RATING ☐

CARDIO EXERCISE	TIME/DISTANCE	NOTES

STRENGTH TRAINING	WT.	SETS	REPS

NUTRITION NOTES

saturday

STRETCHING ☐　DAILY RATING ☐

CARDIO EXERCISE	TIME/DISTANCE	NOTES

STRENGTH TRAINING	WT.	SETS	REPS

NUTRITION NOTES

sunday

STRETCHING ☐   DAILY RATING ☐

CARDIO EXERCISE _____   TIME/DISTANCE _____   NOTES _____

_____   _____   _____
_____   _____   _____
_____   _____   _____

STRENGTH TRAINING	WT.	SETS	REPS
_____			
_____			
_____			
_____			
_____			
_____			
_____			
_____			
_____			
_____			

NUTRITION NOTES

weekly wrap-up

WEEKLY RATING ☐

GOALS: MET _____   EXCEEDED _____   MAYBE NEXT WEEK _____

CARDIO NOTES _____   STRENGTH NOTES _____   **NUTRITION NOTES**

_____   _____
_____   _____
_____   _____
_____   _____
_____   _____
_____   _____
_____   _____
_____   _____
_____   _____

TOTAL CARDIO SESSIONS ☐   TOTAL STRENGTH SESSIONS ☐   TOTAL STRETCHING SESSIONS ☐

Goals: _____
_____

Dates: _____

monday

STRETCHING ☐   DAILY RATING ☐

CARDIO EXERCISE	TIME/DISTANCE	NOTES
_____	_____	_____
_____	_____	_____
_____	_____	_____

STRENGTH TRAINING	WT.	SETS	REPS	NUTRITION NOTES
_____				
_____				
_____				
_____				
_____				
_____				
_____				
_____				
_____				
_____				

tuesday

STRETCHING ☐   DAILY RATING ☐

CARDIO EXERCISE	TIME/DISTANCE	NOTES
_____	_____	_____
_____	_____	_____
_____	_____	_____

STRENGTH TRAINING	WT.	SETS	REPS	NUTRITION NOTES
_____				
_____				
_____				
_____				
_____				
_____				
_____				
_____				
_____				
_____				

RESEARCH REPORT ■ *Use it or lose it: In a one-year study, post-menopausal women who lifted weights twice a week gained almost 1 percent bone mass while those who didn't exercise lost 2.5 percent. The active women improved their balance by 14 percent; the inactive women experienced an 8 percent decline.*

wednesday

STRETCHING ▢   DAILY RATING ▢

CARDIO EXERCISE   TIME/DISTANCE   NOTES

STRENGTH TRAINING   WT.   SETS   REPS

NUTRITION NOTES

thursday

STRETCHING ▢   DAILY RATING ▢

CARDIO EXERCISE   TIME/DISTANCE   NOTES

STRENGTH TRAINING   WT.   SETS   REPS

NUTRITION NOTES

> *"Some people think, 'I reached my goal, what's next—quit?'*
> *After reaching a short-term goal, bring to mind your long-term*
> *goals."*
> Steve Hegg, 1984 Olympic gold medalist, cycling

friday

STRETCHING ☐ DAILY RATING ☐

CARDIO EXERCISE	TIME/DISTANCE	NOTES

STRENGTH TRAINING	WT.	SETS	REPS

NUTRITION NOTES

saturday

STRETCHING ☐ DAILY RATING ☐

CARDIO EXERCISE	TIME/DISTANCE	NOTES

STRENGTH TRAINING	WT.	SETS	REPS

NUTRITION NOTES

sunday

STRETCHING ☐   DAILY RATING ☐

CARDIO EXERCISE	TIME/DISTANCE	NOTES

STRENGTH TRAINING	WT.	SETS	REPS

NUTRITION NOTES

weekly wrap-up

WEEKLY RATING ☐

GOALS: MET _____   EXCEEDED _____   MAYBE NEXT WEEK _____

CARDIO NOTES	STRENGTH NOTES

NUTRITION NOTES

TOTAL CARDIO SESSIONS ☐   TOTAL STRENGTH SESSIONS ☐   TOTAL STRETCHING SESSIONS ☐

Goals: _____

_____

Dates: _____

monday

STRETCHING ☐   DAILY RATING ☐

CARDIO EXERCISE	TIME/DISTANCE	NOTES
_____	_____	_____
_____	_____	_____
_____	_____	_____

STRENGTH TRAINING	WT.	SETS	REPS	NUTRITION NOTES
_____				
_____				
_____				
_____				
_____				
_____				
_____				
_____				
_____				
_____				

tuesday

STRETCHING ☐   DAILY RATING ☐

CARDIO EXERCISE	TIME/DISTANCE	NOTES
_____	_____	_____
_____	_____	_____
_____	_____	_____

STRENGTH TRAINING	WT.	SETS	REPS	NUTRITION NOTES
_____				
_____				
_____				
_____				
_____				
_____				
_____				
_____				
_____				

wednesday

STRETCHING ☐   DAILY RATING ☐

CARDIO EXERCISE   TIME/DISTANCE   NOTES

_____   _____   _____
_____   _____   _____
_____   _____   _____
_____   _____   _____

STRENGTH TRAINING   WT.   SETS   REPS

STRENGTH TRAINING	WT.	SETS	REPS	NUTRITION NOTES
_____				
_____				
_____				
_____				
_____				
_____				
_____				
_____				
_____				
_____				

thursday

STRETCHING ☐   DAILY RATING ☐

CARDIO EXERCISE   TIME/DISTANCE   NOTES

_____   _____   _____
_____   _____   _____
_____   _____   _____

STRENGTH TRAINING   WT.   SETS   REPS

STRENGTH TRAINING	WT.	SETS	REPS	NUTRITION NOTES
_____				
_____				
_____				
_____				
_____				
_____				
_____				
_____				
_____				

"What I enjoy most about training is that it gives you the power to change. Training makes me realize I can change things positively in life." Donna Hawkins, Masters Nordic skiing world champion

friday

STRETCHING ☐   DAILY RATING ☐

CARDIO EXERCISE	TIME/DISTANCE	NOTES

STRENGTH TRAINING	WT.	SETS	REPS	NUTRITION NOTES

saturday

STRETCHING ☐   DAILY RATING ☐

CARDIO EXERCISE	TIME/DISTANCE	NOTES

STRENGTH TRAINING	WT.	SETS	REPS	NUTRITION NOTES

SPORTSPEAK ■ *Wall rats (a.k.a. Rockjocks) (n.): People who spend the better part of their lives hanging from rock walls. Usage: "There's no space left to climb—this place is covered with wall rats!"*

sunday

STRETCHING ☐ DAILY RATING ☐

CARDIO EXERCISE _____ TIME/DISTANCE _____ NOTES _____

STRENGTH TRAINING _____ WT. SETS REPS

NUTRITION NOTES

weekly wrap-up

WEEKLY RATING ☐

GOALS: MET _____ EXCEEDED _____ MAYBE NEXT WEEK _____

CARDIO NOTES _____ STRENGTH NOTES _____

NUTRITION NOTES

TOTAL CARDIO SESSIONS ☐   TOTAL STRENGTH SESSIONS ☐   TOTAL STRETCHING SESSIONS ☐

Goals: _____
_____
_____

Dates: _____
_____

monday

STRETCHING ☐   DAILY RATING ☐

CARDIO EXERCISE	TIME/DISTANCE	NOTES
_____	_____	_____
_____	_____	_____
_____	_____	_____

STRENGTH TRAINING	WT.	SETS	REPS
_____			
_____			
_____			
_____			
_____			
_____			
_____			
_____			
_____			
_____			

NUTRITION NOTES

tuesday

STRETCHING ☐   DAILY RATING ☐

CARDIO EXERCISE	TIME/DISTANCE	NOTES
_____	_____	_____
_____	_____	_____
_____	_____	_____

STRENGTH TRAINING	WT.	SETS	REPS
_____			
_____			
_____			
_____			
_____			
_____			
_____			
_____			
_____			
_____			

NUTRITION NOTES

RESEARCH REPORT ▓ *There's no excuse for bicycling without a helmet. Research shows that helmets have no impact on your body temperature, head skin temperature, sweat rate, or heart rate — but universal helmet use would save one life each day and prevent one head injury every four minutes.*

wednesday

STRETCHING ☐   DAILY RATING ☐

CARDIO EXERCISE	TIME/DISTANCE	NOTES

STRENGTH TRAINING	WT.	SETS	REPS	NUTRITION NOTES

thursday

STRETCHING ☐   DAILY RATING ☐

CARDIO EXERCISE	TIME/DISTANCE	NOTES

STRENGTH TRAINING	WT.	SETS	REPS	NUTRITION NOTES

> *"I come up with a goal in my head, whether it's a specific time or to win a race, and I write it down and tape it to my bathroom mirror so I can see it every morning."*
>
> *Alex Kostich, world Masters record-holder in the 400-meter and 800-meter freestyle and the 400-meter individual medley*

friday

STRETCHING ☐ DAILY RATING ☐

CARDIO EXERCISE   TIME/DISTANCE   NOTES

_____ _____ _____
_____ _____ _____
_____ _____ _____

STRENGTH TRAINING   WT.   SETS   REPS

NUTRITION NOTES

saturday

STRETCHING ☐ DAILY RATING ☐

CARDIO EXERCISE   TIME/DISTANCE   NOTES

_____ _____ _____
_____ _____ _____
_____ _____ _____

STRENGTH TRAINING   WT.   SETS   REPS

NUTRITION NOTES

SPORTSPEAK ■ *Bomb (v.): To ride down a mountain-bike trail at high speed. Usage: "I always bomb that section of the trail."*

sunday

STRETCHING ☐   DAILY RATING ☐

CARDIO EXERCISE	TIME/DISTANCE	NOTES

STRENGTH TRAINING	WT.	SETS	REPS

NUTRITION NOTES

weekly wrap-up

WEEKLY RATING ☐

GOALS: MET _____   EXCEEDED _____   MAYBE NEXT WEEK _____

CARDIO NOTES	STRENGTH NOTES	

NUTRITION NOTES

TOTAL CARDIO SESSIONS ☐   TOTAL STRENGTH SESSIONS ☐   TOTAL STRETCHING SESSIONS ☐

Goals: _____
_____
_____

Dates: _____
_____

monday

STRETCHING ☐ DAILY RATING ☐

CARDIO EXERCISE _____ TIME/DISTANCE _____ NOTES _____

_____ _____ _____

_____ _____ _____

_____ _____ _____

STRENGTH TRAINING _____ WT.　SETS　REPS

			NUTRITION NOTES

tuesday

STRETCHING ☐ DAILY RATING ☐

CARDIO EXERCISE _____ TIME/DISTANCE _____ NOTES _____

_____ _____ _____

_____ _____ _____

_____ _____ _____

STRENGTH TRAINING _____ WT.　SETS　REPS

			NUTRITION NOTES

TRAINING TIP ■ *It's a myth that overweight people should lose pounds before starting to lift weights. Pumping iron can help you lose weight and keep it off by maintaining — and perhaps even speeding up — your metabolism.*

wednesday

STRETCHING ☐   DAILY RATING ☐

CARDIO EXERCISE	TIME/DISTANCE	NOTES

STRENGTH TRAINING	WT.	SETS	REPS

NUTRITION NOTES

thursday

STRETCHING ☐   DAILY RATING ☐

CARDIO EXERCISE	TIME/DISTANCE	NOTES

STRENGTH TRAINING	WT.	SETS	REPS

NUTRITION NOTES

"I let the way I feel each day dictate what activity I do. That way I stay in shape but don't get bored or burned out."

Jim Karn, world-class rock climber

friday

STRETCHING ☐   DAILY RATING ☐

CARDIO EXERCISE	TIME/DISTANCE	NOTES

STRENGTH TRAINING	WT.	SETS	REPS	NUTRITION NOTES

saturday

STRETCHING ☐   DAILY RATING ☐

CARDIO EXERCISE	TIME/DISTANCE	NOTES

STRENGTH TRAINING	WT.	SETS	REPS	NUTRITION NOTES

sunday

STRETCHING ☐   DAILY RATING ☐

CARDIO EXERCISE _____   TIME/DISTANCE _____   NOTES _____

_____   _____   _____
_____   _____   _____
_____   _____   _____

STRENGTH TRAINING _____   WT.   SETS   REPS

NUTRITION NOTES

weekly wrap-up

WEEKLY RATING ☐

GOALS: MET _____   EXCEEDED _____   MAYBE NEXT WEEK _____

CARDIO NOTES _____   STRENGTH NOTES _____   **NUTRITION NOTES**

TOTAL CARDIO SESSIONS ☐   TOTAL STRENGTH SESSIONS ☐   TOTAL STRETCHING SESSIONS ☐

Goals: _____

_____

_____

Dates: _____

monday

STRETCHING ☐   DAILY RATING ☐

CARDIO EXERCISE	TIME/DISTANCE	NOTES
_____	_____	_____
_____	_____	_____
_____	_____	_____

STRENGTH TRAINING	WT.	SETS	REPS	NUTRITION NOTES
_____				
_____				
_____				
_____				
_____				
_____				
_____				
_____				
_____				
_____				
_____				

tuesday

STRETCHING ☐   DAILY RATING ☐

CARDIO EXERCISE	TIME/DISTANCE	NOTES
_____	_____	_____
_____	_____	_____
_____	_____	_____

STRENGTH TRAINING	WT.	SETS	REPS	NUTRITION NOTES
_____				
_____				
_____				
_____				
_____				
_____				
_____				
_____				
_____				
_____				

RESEARCH REPORT ■ *Lifting weights builds self-confidence as well as strength. In a year-long study, women who lifted weights twice a week reported feeling happier, more energetic, and more confident than before.*

wednesday

STRETCHING ☐   DAILY RATING ☐

CARDIO EXERCISE	TIME/DISTANCE	NOTES
_____	_____	_____
_____	_____	_____
_____	_____	_____
_____	_____	_____

STRENGTH TRAINING	WT.	SETS	REPS	
_____				**NUTRITION NOTES**
_____				
_____				
_____				
_____				
_____				
_____				
_____				
_____				

thursday

STRETCHING ☐   DAILY RATING ☐

CARDIO EXERCISE	TIME/DISTANCE	NOTES
_____	_____	_____
_____	_____	_____
_____	_____	_____
_____	_____	_____

STRENGTH TRAINING	WT.	SETS	REPS	
_____				**NUTRITION NOTES**
_____				
_____				
_____				
_____				
_____				
_____				
_____				
_____				

"It's important to have training partners—we challenge and help each other. None of the successful athletes in this sport trains in seclusion." Brian Brown, U.S. national kayak team

friday

STRETCHING ☐ DAILY RATING ☐

CARDIO EXERCISE   TIME/DISTANCE   NOTES

STRENGTH TRAINING   WT.   SETS   REPS

NUTRITION NOTES

saturday

STRETCHING ☐ DAILY RATING ☐

CARDIO EXERCISE   TIME/DISTANCE   NOTES

STRENGTH TRAINING   WT.   SETS   REPS

NUTRITION NOTES

sunday

STRETCHING ☐   DAILY RATING ☐

CARDIO EXERCISE _____   TIME/DISTANCE _____   NOTES _____

_____   _____   _____

_____   _____   _____

_____   _____   _____

STRENGTH TRAINING   WT.   SETS   REPS

_____

_____

_____

_____

_____

_____

_____

_____

NUTRITION NOTES

weekly wrap-up

WEEKLY RATING ☐

GOALS: MET _____   EXCEEDED _____   MAYBE NEXT WEEK _____

CARDIO NOTES _____   STRENGTH NOTES _____

NUTRITION NOTES

TOTAL CARDIO SESSIONS ☐   TOTAL STRENGTH SESSIONS ☐   TOTAL STRETCHING SESSIONS ☐

23

Goals:

Dates:

monday

STRETCHING ☐   DAILY RATING ☐

CARDIO EXERCISE	TIME/DISTANCE	NOTES

STRENGTH TRAINING	WT.	SETS	REPS	NUTRITION NOTES

tuesday

STRETCHING ☐   DAILY RATING ☐

CARDIO EXERCISE	TIME/DISTANCE	NOTES

STRENGTH TRAINING	WT.	SETS	REPS	NUTRITION NOTES

TRAINING TIP ■ *Never wear clothing designed to help you lose weight by sweating away the pounds — you could become seriously dehydrated. Besides, any weight you lose by wearing this type of clothing is water, not fat. You'll gain it right back when you replenish the lost fluids.*

wednesday

STRETCHING ☐   DAILY RATING ☐

CARDIO EXERCISE	TIME/DISTANCE	NOTES

STRENGTH TRAINING	WT.	SETS	REPS	NUTRITION NOTES

thursday

STRETCHING ☐   DAILY RATING ☐

CARDIO EXERCISE	TIME/DISTANCE	NOTES

STRENGTH TRAINING	WT.	SETS	REPS	NUTRITION NOTES

"Never stop believing in yourself."

Johnny G, creator of the Spinning® cycling program and finisher, Race Across AMerica

friday

STRETCHING ☐   DAILY RATING ☐

CARDIO EXERCISE	TIME/DISTANCE	NOTES

STRENGTH TRAINING	WT.	SETS	REPS

NUTRITION NOTES

saturday

STRETCHING ☐   DAILY RATING ☐

CARDIO EXERCISE	TIME/DISTANCE	NOTES

STRENGTH TRAINING	WT.	SETS	REPS

NUTRITION NOTES

sunday

STRETCHING ☐   DAILY RATING ☐

CARDIO EXERCISE   TIME/DISTANCE   NOTES

STRENGTH TRAINING   WT.   SETS   REPS   **NUTRITION NOTES**

weekly wrap-up

WEEKLY RATING ☐

GOALS: MET _____   EXCEEDED _____   MAYBE NEXT WEEK _____

CARDIO NOTES   STRENGTH NOTES   **NUTRITION NOTES**

TOTAL CARDIO SESSIONS ☐   TOTAL STRENGTH SESSIONS ☐   TOTAL STRETCHING SESSIONS ☐

Goals:

Dates:

monday

STRETCHING ☐   DAILY RATING ☐

CARDIO EXERCISE	TIME/DISTANCE	NOTES

STRENGTH TRAINING	WT.	SETS	REPS	NUTRITION NOTES

tuesday

STRETCHING ☐   DAILY RATING ☐

CARDIO EXERCISE	TIME/DISTANCE	NOTES

STRENGTH TRAINING	WT.	SETS	REPS	NUTRITION NOTES

wednesday

STRETCHING ☐   DAILY RATING ☐

CARDIO EXERCISE   TIME/DISTANCE   NOTES

STRENGTH TRAINING   WT.   SETS   REPS   **NUTRITION NOTES**

thursday

STRETCHING ☐   DAILY RATING ☐

CARDIO EXERCISE   TIME/DISTANCE   NOTES

STRENGTH TRAINING   WT.   SETS   REPS   **NUTRITION NOTES**

> **"When you look back at your log and see all the work you've done, give yourself a pat on the back and say, 'Yeah, I'm fit.'"**
>
> *Matt Giusto, 1996 Olympian, 5,000-meter run*

friday

STRETCHING ☐   DAILY RATING ☐

CARDIO EXERCISE	TIME/DISTANCE	NOTES

STRENGTH TRAINING	WT.	SETS	REPS

NUTRITION NOTES

saturday

STRETCHING ☐   DAILY RATING ☐

CARDIO EXERCISE	TIME/DISTANCE	NOTES

STRENGTH TRAINING	WT.	SETS	REPS

NUTRITION NOTES

sunday

STRETCHING ☐   DAILY RATING ☐

CARDIO EXERCISE _____   TIME/DISTANCE _____   NOTES _____

_____ _____ _____
_____ _____ _____
_____ _____ _____

STRENGTH TRAINING _____   WT.   SETS   REPS

NUTRITION NOTES

weekly wrap-up

WEEKLY RATING ☐

GOALS: MET _____   EXCEEDED _____   MAYBE NEXT WEEK _____

CARDIO NOTES _____   STRENGTH NOTES _____   **NUTRITION NOTES**

TOTAL CARDIO SESSIONS ☐   TOTAL STRENGTH SESSIONS ☐   TOTAL STRETCHING SESSIONS ☐

How Many Calories Do You Burn?

This chart provides an estimate of the number of calories you'll burn per hour doing different activities. Keep in mind that the numbers vary depending on your weight, metabolism, and muscle mass.

	CALORIES BURNED PER HOUR	
ACTIVITY	135-POUND PERSON	180-POUND PERSON
Aerobic dance		
moderate intensity	329	443
high intensity	549	738
Basketball (not counting breaks)	512	689
Bicycling (outdoors)		
12 mph	483	649
15 mph	604	812
18 mph	725	974
Golf (no cart)	293	394
Running		
10-minute miles	589	877
9-minute miles	718	965
8-minute miles	800	1,075
7-minute miles	905	1,216
Rowing	392	526
Swimming		
crawl, 35 yards/minute	396	528
crawl, 50 yards/minute	570	768
breaststroke, 30 yards/minute	384	516
breaststroke, 40 yards/minute	516	690
Tennis		
singles	399	536
doubles	146	197
Walking		
20-minute miles	211	284
15-minute miles	260	350
Circuit weight training (not including rest)	439	590

Workout Ratings: The Big Picture

At the end of each week, record your daily and weekly ratings here. This chart will help you see weekly and monthly patterns in your training. You might notice, for instance, that you perform better when you rest two days rather than one or when you take one extra-easy week each month. If you get injured, a glance at your chart might help explain why.

WEEK	M	T	W	T	F	S	S	WEEKLY
1								
2								
3								
4								
5								
6								
7								
8								
9								
10								
11								
12								
13								
14								
15								
16								
17								
18								
19								
20								
21								
22								
23								
24								

Personal Records

Don't think that the only place to set a record is in a competition. Use this chart to log breakthroughs in your workouts—whether it's the first time you bench-press 120 pounds, cycle 50 miles, or exercise five times in one week.

DATE	ACTIVITY	ACCOMPLISHMENT

Six-month Wrap-up

Congrats! You've completed your log. Before you start your next diary, take some time to see what you've accomplished over the last six months. Did you meet your goals? Jotting down the answer here will help you set new ones.

■ **Overall goals**
_____
_____
_____
_____

■ **Cardio exercise goals**
_____
_____
_____
_____

■ **Strength-training goals**
_____
_____
_____
_____

■ **Nutrition goals**
_____
_____
_____
_____

resources

These books can expand your knowledge of topics covered in this book.

General Fitness

The Complete Home Fitness Handbook, Ed Burke. Champaign, Ill.: Human Kinetics, 1996

Fitness for Dummies, Suzanne Schlosberg and Liz Neporent, M.A. Foster City, Calif.: IDG Books Worldwide, 1996

Weight Training

The Complete Book of Abs and *The Complete Book of Butt and Legs*, Kurt Brungardt. NY: Villard, 1993 and 1995, respectively

Weight Training for Dummies, Liz Neporent, M.A., and Suzanne Schlosberg. Foster City, Calif.: IDG Books Worldwide, 1997

A Woman's Book of Strength, Karen Andes. NY: The Berkley Publishing Group, 1995

Injury Treatment and Prevention

The Return to Glory Days, Morton Dean and Benjamin Gelfand, P.T. NY: Pocket Books, 1997

Sports Nutrition

High Performance Nutrition, Susan Kleiner and Maggie Greenwood-Robinson. NY: John Wiley & Sons, 1996

Nancy Clark's Sports Nutrition Guidebook, Second Edition, Nancy Clark. Champaign, Ill.: Human Kinetics, 1996

Nutrition for Women: The Complete Guide, Elizabeth Somer. NY: Henry Holt, 1993

sources

The following are the sources for the Research Report items.

Week 2

David C. Nieman, "Physical activity and immune function in elderly women," *Medicine & Science in Sports & Exercise* 25 (July 1993): 823–31.

Week 4

A. C. King, "Moderate-intensity exercise and self-rated quality of sleep in older adults," *Journal of the American Medical Association* 277 (January 1, 1997): 32–37.

Week 6

M. A. Fiatarone, "High-intensity strength training in nonagenarians: Effects on skeletal muscle," *Journal of the American Medical Association* 263 (June 13, 1990): 3029–34.

Week 8

Marie H. Murphy and Adrianne E. Hardman, "Brisk walking in women: short versus long bouts," *Medicine & Science in Sports & Exercise* (January 1998) 152–56.

Week 10

S. N. Blair, "Changes in physical fitness and all-cause mortality: a prospective study of healthy and unhealthy men," *Journal of the American Medical Association* 273 (April 12, 1995): 1093–98.

Week 12

M. L. Skender, "Comparison of 2-year weight loss trends in behavioral treatments of obesity: diet, exercise, and combination interventions," *Journal of the American Dietetic Association* 96 (April 1996): 342–46.

Week 14

J. P. Wallace, "Twelve month adherence of adults who joined a fitness program with a spouse vs. without a spouse," *Journal of Sports Medicine and Physical Fitness* 35 (September 1995): 206–13.

Week 16

A. A. Hakim, "Effects of walking on mortality among nonsmoking retired men." *New England Journal of Medicine* 33 (January 8, 1998): 94–99.

Week 18

Miriam Nelson, "Effects of high-intensity strength training on multiple factors for osteoporotic fractures," *Journal of the American Medical Association* 272 (1994): 1909–14.

Week 20

Melinda Sheffield-Moore, "Thermoregulatory responses to cycling with and without a helmet," *Medicine & Science in Sports & Exercise* 29 (June 1997): 755–61.

Week 22

Miriam E. Nelson, *Strong Women Stay Young* (New York: Bantam Books, 1997), pp. 11–13.

Week 24

Owen Anderson, "Extra Miles and Workouts Don't Help Novice Marathoners," *Running Research News* 11 (March 1995).

acknowledgments

I'm most grateful to Brad Kearns and Petit Pinson, who went way above and beyond the call of duty. Thanks, guys!

Thanks also to Marnie Cochran, my editor, who believed in this book from the start, and to Liz Neporent, who's always willing to share her expertise. As usual, Nancy Gottesman gets credit for listening to me kvetch. So does my loving family.

I also appreciate the help of Richard Motzkin and the athletes who agreed to be quoted in the book, along with those who contributed the Sportspeak items: Brian Anastasio, Eloise Brown, Christian Cabanilla, Atom Crawford, Darren Darsey, Ian Farquar, Donna Freund, Tina Gerson, Alex Kostich, Kay Kudo, Courtney Lowe, Melanie Sarko, Anthony Pinson, Geoff Schott, Matthew Schott, Dave Talskey, Blair Whitney, and Heidi Whitney.